Pediatric and
Adolescent AIDS

Dedicated with love and affection to our families
Cindy, Jay, and Lee—SH
Julie, Jennifer, and Stephany—GM
Lynne and Nicholas—JR

Pediatric and Adolescent AIDS

Research Findings
From the Social Sciences

Scott W. Henggeler
Gary B. Melton
James R. Rodrigue

SAGE Publications
International Educational and Professional Publisher
Newbury Park   London   New Delhi

For information address:

SAGE Publications, Inc.
2455 Teller Road
Newbury Park, California 91320

SAGE Publications Ltd.
6 Bonhill Street
London EC2A 4PU
United Kingdom

SAGE Publications India Pvt. Ltd.
M-32 Market
Greater Kailash I
New Delhi 110 048 India

Printed in the United States of America

Library of Congress Cataloging-in-Publication Data

Henggeler, Scott W.
   Pediatric and adolescent AIDS: research findings from the social sciences / Scott W. Henggeler, Gary B. Melton, James R. Rodrigue.
        p.   cm.
   Includes bibliographical references and index.
   ISBN 0-8039-3982-5 (cl.).   — ISBN 0-8039-3983-3 (pb)
   1. AIDS (Disease) in children.   2. AIDS (Disease) in children—
Social aspects.   3. AIDS (Disease) in adolescence.   4. AIDS
(Disease) in adolescence—Social aspects.   5. Risk-taking
(Psychology) in adolescence.   I. Melton, Gary B.   II. Rodrigue,
James R.   III. Title.
   [DNLM: 1. Aquired Immunodeficiency Syndrome—epidemiology.
2. Acquired Immunodeficiency Syndrome—in adolescence.   3. Aquired
Immunodeficiency Syndrome—in infants & childhood. WD 308 H511p]
RJ387.A25H46   1992
618.92'9792—dc20   92-13382

92 93 94 95   10 9 8 7 6 5 4 3 2 1

Sage Production Editor: Tara S. Mead

Contents

Preface

The incidence of HIV infection and AIDS among infants, children, adolescents, and childbearing women has risen sharply in recent years, and epidemiological evidence indicates that this trend will continue. Unlike most other diseases of childhood, AIDS progresses rapidly and leads to death in all instances. It has the unique possibility of affecting and eventually killing more than one family member at the same time. Children and adolescents with AIDS experience a vast range of acute and chronic illnesses that demand intensive outpatient and inpatient medical services. Indeed, frequent illness and hospitalization may represent insurmountable social and psychological challenges to those children and families whose coping resources are limited.

This book reviews AIDS-related studies that pertain to children and adolescents. The pediatric and adolescent AIDS literature is truly multidisciplinary, with important research being conducted across multiple areas of the social sciences and the biological sciences. The authors of this volume were selected because of their special expertise in areas that are especially germane to the study of pediatric and adolescent AIDS (e.g., behavior problems in adolescence, ethics and the law, pediatric medicine). To the best of our knowledge, this volume is the first to integrate a substantive body of empirical research in the area of pediatric and adolescent AIDS.

Introductory chapters provide the reader with a concise overview of the virology, immunology, clinical features, and epidemiology of pediatric and adolescent AIDS. Such knowledge provides a fundamental background for social science research in the area. Chapter 3 reviews the emerging literature on youths' AIDS knowledge and attitudes and the associations between such cognitive variables and risk-taking behavior. Chapters 4 and 5 examine extant research regarding adolescent sexual behavior and intravenous drug use, respectively, as well as the psychosocial correlates of such risk-taking behaviors. Together, knowledge gained from these literatures has important implications for the development of preventive programs, as described in Chapter 6, which also discusses current medical treatments.

In Chapter 7, significant attention is devoted to the many complex legal and ethical problems associated with AIDS, especially as they concern pediatric and adolescent populations. Finally, Chapter 8 includes suggestions for future research across a range of pertinent topics. Pediatric and adolescent AIDS is a rapidly emerging area of research, and we hope that this volume facilitates the work of researchers and provides students and clinicians with an empirically-based understanding of key issues.

ONE

Virology, Immunology, and Clinical Features

Ryan White

Seven-year-old Nicholas lives in a small rural community with his mother, father, and 9-year-old sister. A normally developing second grader, Nicholas is bright, popular, highly regarded by his teacher, and active in Cub Scouts. Indeed, it would appear that Nicholas is living a normal childhood, despite the fact that he has hemophilia. Within a few days, however, his experience of a normal childhood is shattered, and in its place is erected a world of hatred, betrayal, prejudice, and social isolation.

Nicholas tests positive for the human immunodeficiency virus (HIV), the etiologic agent of acquired immunodeficiency syndrome (AIDS). His parents decide not to tell school administrators about the diagnosis and send him to school as usual. Upon arriving at school, however, Nicholas is greeted at the front door by the principal, who tells him he cannot enter. Nicholas sits tearfully alone outside the school while the principal calls Nicholas's mother to retrieve him. The principal informs Nicholas's mother that he has learned "through the grapevine" that her son has AIDS, and therefore he will not permit Nicholas to attend his school. Nicholas remains alone outside the school for 45 minutes until his mother picks him up. The headline in the following morning's newspaper reads, "Boy With

1

AIDS Not Allowed in School." Nicholas's HIV status is no longer a secret.

The principal's decision is upheld by the school board, and for 2 months Nicholas remains at home. All homebound instructors in the area are reportedly unavailable to provide educational instruction. Nicholas's mother is forced to quit her job. His sister is ridiculed by peers at school. Most parents no longer permit their children to play with Nicholas. It takes 2 months for the justice system to overturn the school board's decision and to allow Nicholas to attend school once again. Unfortunately, he continues to be the object of fear, betrayal, and hatred. A third of his peers are not permitted by their parents to attend school if Nicholas is present. Many of those who do attend call him names and have been instructed by their parents not to play with him. Adults also seem to shy away from him. On one occasion during recess, Nicholas falls to the ground and cuts his arm. The teacher on playground duty ushers the other children into the school and tells Nicholas to remain outside while she calls his mother. His mother arrives 15 minutes later to find Nicholas alone on the playground with an injury that has gone untreated. His family moves to a nearby city, but the reception they receive is anything but friendly. Nicholas continues to be isolated socially and withdrawn. His physical health eventually deteriorates, and he dies 2 years later.

In another community, Laura, a young woman with a history of intravenous (IV) drug use, gives birth to her first child. Soon after giving birth, Laura learns that she is HIV infected. Sixteen months later, Laura's child also tests positive for the virus. Laura is informed that any additional offspring will be at significantly high risk for HIV infection. She has two more children, both subsequently testing positive for HIV. Although her children are given free medical services, Laura is unable to receive necessary medication and medical treatment because she refuses to apply for Medicaid. Instead, she is suspected of taking her children's antiviral medications. Her oldest child develops AIDS symptomatology and dies several months later. Laura's health progressively deteriorates, and her children are removed from her care and placed in separate foster homes.

Unfortunately, the two scenarios described above are commonplace, occurring with some variation in hundreds of communities across the United States. Indeed, AIDS is killing our children and youth at a phenomenal pace. It is presently the 9th leading cause of death among children 1 to 4 years of age, the 12th among children 5 to 14 years old, and the 7th in youth between 15 and 24 years of age (Oxtoby, 1991). Moreover, between 5,000 and 10,000 more children and adolescents in the United States are estimated to be infected with HIV (Centers for Disease Control [CDC], 1990a; Oxtoby, 1991). At the present rate of HIV infection, AIDS soon will become one of the top five leading causes of death among infants, children, and adolescents.

Since the first description of AIDS in 1981, rapid advances have been made in understanding the etiology, pathogenesis, and clinical parameters of disease associated with HIV and AIDS in children and adolescents. In recent years, it has become increasingly clear that the development of the HIV pandemic, its diagnosis, and its clinical course in children differ from the patterns observed in adults. An understanding of the medical aspects of HIV infection and AIDS in children and adolescents is important for several reasons. As highlighted above and as further described in Chapter 3, inaccurate information or a poor understanding of the pathophysiology of HIV infection and AIDS may contribute to misconceptions about those who are affected. Furthermore, knowledge of medical features serves as an important backdrop to understanding the physical, social, and psychological stressors affecting children with AIDS and their families. This introductory chapter sets out to describe the virologic and immunologic characteristics, diagnosis, classification, and clinical parameters of HIV infection and AIDS in infants, children, and adolescents.

Virology and Immunology of HIV

HIV is a human retrovirus that carries its genetic code as RNA (ribonucleic acid) and replicates by producing and inserting a DNA (deoxyribonucleic acid) copy of its genetic code into a host cell. Thus genetic information flows in a reverse direction (RNA to DNA rather than DNA to RNA) from that which occurs in most other biological systems. This process involving the RNA-dependent, DNA polymerase is often referred to as *reverse transcriptase*. Researchers have known for years that retroviruses cause cancer and progressive neurological disease in animal models (Teich, 1985). In addition to HIV, however, only two other human retroviruses have been identified: human T-cell lymphotropic virus-type 1 (HTLV-1) and human immunodeficiency virus-type 2 (HIV-2). HTLV-1, the first human retrovirus to be discovered (Wong-Staal & Gallo, 1985), is an etiologic agent in certain types of cancer (T-cell lymphoma) and neurological disease (spastic paraparesis). HIV-2 is a more recent discovery and may be quite similar to HIV in its biological properties and consequent symptomatology (McClure & Weiss, 1987; Weber & Weiss, 1988). All three human retroviruses are members of the retrovirus subfamily called *lentiviruses*, which are characterized by chronic protracted clinical diseases with generally long incubation periods.

Two single strands of RNA and RNA-dependent, DNA polymerase constitute the core of HIV. Also, within its RNA genome, HIV contains structural proteins, enzymes necessary for reverse transcription, and regulatory proteins that determine the pathogenesis and rate of viral replication (Haseltine & Wong-Staal, 1988; McCutchan, 1990). The viral membrane (outer envelope) is acquired from the host cell as the virus exits through the cell membrane.

The HIV life cycle involves several complex stages leading to the reproduction of numerous viral cells (progeny) within the host cell. These steps consist of (a) HIV binding to a cellular receptor; (b) the virus entering the host cell; (c) cellular enzymes breaking the virus into its components; (d) viral RNA being transcribed into DNA (reverse transcriptase); (e) viral DNA being integrated into the cell genome; (f) viral DNA being transcribed back to RNA, which is then translated into viral proteins; and (g) formation and budding of new virus particles that exit through the host cell membrane (Sattentau, 1990). The host cell subsequently dies.

A necessary condition for viral infection and replication is a permissive cellular receptor. The receptor for HIV is the CD4 (cluster determinant) molecule, which is central to most immunologic reactions. Virtually all cells expressing this antigen on their surface are vulnerable to HIV infection, including the helper subset of human T lymphocytes (T4), monocytes/macrophages, some B lymphocytes, and possibly glial cells (Ho, Pomerantz, & Kaplan, 1987; Stiehm & Wara, 1991; Weber & Weiss, 1988). Because the functioning of many other cells in the immune system is dependent on CD4 lymphocytes, the loss of CD4 T helper cells is responsible for many of the immunological aberrations that are seen in children with HIV infection. These abnormalities include greater susceptibility to opportunistic infection, bacterial infections, and an increased propensity toward malignancy, lymphoid interstitial pneumonitis, and thrombocytopenia (Stiehm & Wara, 1991). Thus HIV infects and destroys the very cell that is designed for protection against viral infection.

Another subset of T lymphocytes that plays a key role in mediating cytotoxicity and suppression is the T8 cell, which is defined by the cell surface antigen CD8. Indeed, in addition to using CD4 depletion as an index of immunologic deterioration, researchers and clinicians have used the ratio of CD4 to CD8 antigens as an immunologic marker (McNamara, 1989; Rosenberg & Fauci, 1991; Stiehm & Wara, 1991). Early research, for example, determined that individuals infected with HIV demonstrated a dramatic reduction in the absolute number of circulating T4 cells and very little change in the number of T8 cells, thus resulting in an inverted T4:T8 ratio. Although these two immunologic markers are usually related to the course of illness, there are notable exceptions. For instance, severe clinical illness (e.g., severe opportunistic infection in children, Kaposi's sarcoma in adults) has been reported in the absence of CD4 depletion, and the utility of the CD4:CD8 ratio seems to vary depending on age (McNamara, 1989; Stiehm & Wara, 1991).

One intriguing immunologic finding is that the rapid CD4 depletion occurs despite the fact that only a very small percentage of CD4 cells is actually infected (Stiehm & Wara, 1991). The mechanism by which the formation and function of uninfected CD4 cells are affected remains unclear. Several possible explanations, however, have been advanced: HIV might infect CD4 cells at very early stages of development, thus not allowing them to mature fully; infected CD4 cells might yield toxic substances that would affect the development and function of other CD4 cells; or infected CD4 cells might not produce factors necessary for the complete maturation of T4 lymphocyte cells (Stiehm & Wara, 1991).

Although the virologic and immunologic abnormalities seen in young children with AIDS are generally similar to those observed in adolescents and young adults, there are important distinctions. First, unlike adults (or even children and adolescents with hemophilia), vertically infected children—those born to HIV-infected mothers—have an immature immune system that is less able to resist infection. Consequently, they have a briefer incubation period and a more rapid, fulminant disease process. It has been suggested that the difference between young children and adults in the rate of disease progression is due to the timing of HIV infection in utero (Rosenberg & Fauci, 1991). If HIV infection occurs concurrent with

rapid expansion of normal CD4 cells in the fetus, the normal migra-
tion of these cells through the bone marrow, spleen, and thymus
could result in the rapid spread of HIV throughout the body.

Second, the initial immunologic marker in infants and young
children is abnormal B-cell function (e.g., elevated numbers of B
cells, hypergammaglobulinemia) with relatively normal T-cell immunity (Nadal et al., 1989). These abnormalities in B-cell immunity
predispose infants and children to more severe bacterial infections
than those seen in adults. In one study, Bernstein, Krieger, Novick,
Sicklick, and Rubinstein (1985) found that more than 50% of HIV-
infected infants and children experienced at least one serious bacterial infection. Moreover, young children are more likely to die from
serious bacterial, rather than opportunistic, infection.

Third, there is evidence to suggest that children with HIV infection may not present with the same degree of CD4 depletion as
adults. Shannon and Ammann (1985), for instance, noted that many
infants and children with HIV infection manifest normal total lymphocyte counts and that approximately 15% of infected children
have normal CD4:CD8 ratios. Severe opportunistic infection, however, can occur even in the face of normal CD4 numbers.

Detection and Progression of HIV

Assays of Immunological Functioning

Ideally, culture or antigen detection methods are used to detect
the actual presence of HIV in blood or tissues. Nonetheless, the presence of HIV antibodies in the serum is often used as evidence of HIV
exposure, because the availability and sensitivity of some diagnostic
methods are limited. This detection method has limited validity in
infants. Infants who are HIV infected may appear normal initially
and may exhibit no specific signs of illness. Likewise, the presence
of maternal antibodies in the infant's blood may erroneously lead
to antibody-positive test results for up to 18 months following birth,
and, in some cases, antibody-negative results may be obtained even
though HIV has been cultured from the infant's blood (Mok et al.,
1987; European Collaborative Study, 1988).

Several immunological tests are used to detect HIV or HIV antibodies from blood, cerebrospinal fluid (CSF), or other bodily fluids.

Previously discussed immunologic parameters typically are part of the diagnostic battery. The use of classic immunologic abnormalities —low CD4 counts, elevated CD8 counts, reversed CD4:CD8 ratio, elevated immunoglobulin levels, and decreased specific antibody responses—has greater diagnostic utility for adults than for infants and young children, because little prospective data are available on these younger samples. Assays of circulating p24 are also used to detect HIV in the blood, although they are not very sensitive during the early stages of infection and are used primarily to monitor the course of infection (Rogers et al., 1989).

Two of the more promising assays for detecting HIV are the polymerase chain reaction (PCR) test (Edwards et al., 1989; Ou et al., 1988; Rogers et al., 1989) and the in-vitro antibody production (IVAP) assay (Amadori et al., 1988). PCR is considered a major diagnostic breakthrough because it allows for the detection of a very small amount of latent virus from months to years prior to the detection of HIV antibodies. PCR also may turn out to be the most useful diagnostic test for infants because (a) it detects HIV itself rather than HIV antibodies and consequently cannot be confounded by the presence of maternal antibodies; (b) unlike most other assays, it requires only a very small amount of blood; and (c) testing can be completed in one day, thus permitting immediate medical intervention. Although the sensitivity, specificity, and limitations of PCR are as yet unknown, recent studies highlight its prospective utility. Rogers et al. (1989), for example, found that PCR accurately detected HIV infection in about 60% of infants who were tested during the neonatal period. IVAP, which detects the presence of antibody-producing B lymphocytes, also avoids the problem of persistent maternal antibodies; however, it is not yet clear how well this test identifies infected infants during the neonatal period (Rogers, Ou, Kilbourne, & Schochetman, 1991).

When the virus itself cannot be isolated, laboratory techniques are used to detect antibodies to the virus. The diagnostic test used most frequently for the detection of antibodies to HIV is the enzyme-linked immunosorbent assay (ELISA), which isolates circulating HIV antibodies that are reactive to purified viral lysate. Despite its reportedly high accuracy and sensitivity, ELISA is not diagnostically helpful during the period of time (4 to 6 weeks, or occasionally much longer) it takes for HIV antibodies to develop in adolescents and adults (Schumacher, Garrett, Tegmeier, & Thomas, 1988). Consequently, false positives and false negatives occur with ELISAs, though false positive results are more common (Wilber, 1990).

Because of the low specificity of ELISA, the use of supplementary tests is considered mandatory in confirming HIV infection. Indeed, individuals are not typically informed of their laboratory findings until supplemental tests are conducted (CDC, 1987b). Commonly used supplemental laboratory methods include immunoelectrophoresis procedures (e.g., Western Blot), immunofluorescence assay (IFA), and radioimmunoprecipitation assay (RIPA). The CDC (1987b) reports that the combined false positive rate for ELISA and the Western Blot is 1:100; it may take up to 6 months for the host body to produce enough HIV antibodies for either of the two tests to detect their presence (Ranki, Valle, & Krohn, 1987). Unfortunately, the presence of HIV antibodies does not mean that one has protection from developing AIDS symptoms, but that one has been exposed to HIV and now can transmit the virus to others even while showing no overt evidence of illness. Moreover, the presence of HIV antibodies does not necessarily mean that one has AIDS; indeed, some individuals remain healthy in all other respects.

As previously noted, conventional tests for antibodies to HIV are not always diagnostically useful for vertically infected infants, because their antibodies cannot be distinguished from those acquired from the mother in utero. Weiblen and her colleagues (Weiblen, Schumacher, & Hoff, 1990; Weiblen et al., 1990), however, have recently documented that HIV infection in infants as young as 6 months can be reliably diagnosed before the onset of symptoms by assaying IgA HIV antibodies after removing IgG antibodies with recombinant protein G. Although maternal IgG HIV antibodies can persist for up to 18 months in infants, IgA HIV antibodies do not cross the placenta. Therefore, IgA may be a useful tool in the early diagnosis of HIV infection in infants. Additional research is necessary to determine if this diagnostic method is as sensitive as others.

More recently, attention has focused on the applicability of amniocentesis, chorionic villus sampling, and percutaneous umbilical blood sampling (i.e., cordocentesis) in the prenatal diagnosis of fetal HIV infection (Landers & Sweet, 1991). Although these procedures hold promise for the future, they presently lack important information about reliability and specificity. Furthermore, the risk of infecting an otherwise healthy fetus with maternal HIV-infected blood seems quite high even with the present technology.

TABLE 1.1   CDC Definition of HIV Infection in Children Under 13
Years of Age

I. Children under 15 months of age with vertical infection must meet one of the
following criteria:
   a. HIV in blood or tissues;
   b. Presence of HIV antibody *and* evidence of both cellular and humoral immune deficiency *and* evidence of symptomatic infection; or
   c. Symptoms meeting previously published CDC case definition for pediatric
AIDS.
II. Older children with vertical infection and children with HIV infection acquired
through other transmission modes must meet one of the following criteria:
   a. HIV in blood or tissues;
   b. Presence of HIV antibody regardless of whether immunologic abnormalities
or symptoms are present; or
   c. Symptoms meeting previously published CDC case definition for pediatric
AIDS.

Definition and Classification

Shortly after the first pediatric and adult AIDS cases were described,
the CDC (1982) created a working epidemiological definition to monitor trends regarding this previously unrecognized immunodeficiency disorder. According to this initial definition, to receive an AIDS
diagnosis a patient had to have a diagnosed opportunistic infection
or malignancy with a cellular immunodeficiency etiology. Patients
with congenital immunodeficiency or viral infection, with previous
immunodeficiency-linked illness, or currently receiving immunosuppressive pharmacotherapy were excluded from this definition. Following extensive case reports of AIDS-related infection in children
in the absence of opportunistic disease (Oleske et al., 1983; Rubinstein
et al., 1983) and the discovery of HIV in 1983, the CDC (1985a) broadened its description of AIDS and included specific diagnostic criteria for children. The 1985 revision also described lymphoid interstitial pneumonitis (or pulmonary lymphoid hyperplasia), a type of
pneumonia considered diagnostic of pediatric AIDS. Finally, the
CDC (1987a) produced its present surveillance case definition for
HIV infection and AIDS, which includes (a) a description of the immunologic deficits seen predominantly in children with HIV infection,
and (b) more stringent HIV diagnostic criteria for children less than
15 months of age, because of the presence of maternal antibodies for
several months following birth (see Table 1.1).

TABLE 1.2   CDC Classification of HIV Infection in Children

Class P-0: Indeterminate Infection
Class P-1: Asymptomatic Infection
    Subclass A: Normal immune functioning
    Subclass B: Abnormal immune functioning (e.g., hypergammaglobulinemia, T4
               lymphopenia, decreased T4:T8 ratio)
    Subclass C: Immune functioning not tested
Class P-2: Symptomatic Infection
    Subclass A: Nonspecific findings (e.g., fever, failure to thrive, recurrent diarrhea,
               generalized lymphadenopathy)
    Subclass B: Progressive neurological disease (e.g., loss of developmental mile-
               stones or intellectual ability, progressive motor deficits)
    Subclass C: Lymphoid interstitial pneumonitis
    Subclass D: Secondary infectious diseases
        Category D-1: Opportunistic infections specified in CDC AIDS surveillance
                   definition
        Category D-2: Unexplained, recurrent serious bacterial infections
        Category D-3: Other specified secondary infectious diseases
    Subclass E: Secondary cancers
        Category E-1: Specified secondary cancers listed in CDC AIDS surveillance
                   definition (e.g., Kaposi's sarcoma, B-cell non-Hodgkin's
                   lymphoma)
        Category E-2: Other cancers possibly secondary to HIV infection
    Subclass F: Other diseases possibly attributable to HIV infections (e.g., hepatitis,
               cardiopathy, hematologic disorders)

In the same year, the CDC (1987a) proposed a classification system for HIV in children under 13 years of age (Table 1.2). Class P-0 includes children up to 15 months of age who were born to infected mothers but who lack definitive evidence of HIV infection or AIDS. Class P-1 and Class P-2 include children without or with previous signs and symptoms, respectively. This classification system, which is used primarily in epidemiological studies and disease surveillance, differs from the classification scheme used for adults. Specifically, for adults there is a fourth category between the asymptomatic and symptomatic stages for those who manifest clinical symptoms of AIDS-related complex (ARC), including severe weight loss or chronic lymphadenopathy in the absence of opportunistic infections. The omission of this fourth category probably reflects the rapid progression of disease in young children, although some have argued that this has led to an underestimate of the number of HIV-infected children who are symptomatic (Grossman, 1988).

Ammann (1990) has suggested the use of a different classification scheme that is based largely on the World Health Organization's classification of immunodeficiency disorders. The scheme states that pediatric AIDS should be diagnosed if the child has (a) a history of a risk factor, (b) laboratory evidence of immunodeficiency, and (c) evidence of HIV infection or antibodies to the virus after 6 months of age. Note that this definition, unlike that used by CDC, does not require documentation of opportunistic infection. Ammann advocates the use of this definition because it allows for early diagnosis of pediatric HIV infection and early initiation of prophylactic therapies. He notes that categorizing children based entirely on stages of symptomatic HIV disease is not useful, because HIV infection progresses so rapidly in infants. Regardless of the definition used, diagnosing HIV infection or AIDS before the onset of opportunistic infection is critical if complications are to be prevented or if life is to be prolonged.

Clinical Manifestations of Pediatric AIDS

The clinical manifestations of AIDS in vertically infected children differ markedly from those observed in adults. For example, the asymptomatic or latency period following HIV infection is much briefer in children than in adults. In adults, HIV antibodies are activated 8 to 12 weeks after initial infection, with rare instances of seroconversion occurring only several months or years after infection (Imagawa et al., 1989). An asymptomatic period lasting months to years typically follows seroconversion. The median latency period between initial exposure to HIV and the onset of clinical symptoms in adults is approximately 10 years (Bacchetti & Moss, 1989; Munoz et al., 1989). In contrast to its initial presentation in adults, HIV in children who are vertically infected tends to have a rather brief incubation period, which is attributable to the infant's inability to produce sufficient levels of HIV antibodies in the absence of maternal antibodies. The median incubation period is estimated at 8 to 10 months (Krasinski, Borkowsky, & Holzman, 1989; Rogers et al., 1987).

Another distinction between vertically acquired HIV and HIV in adults is the greater heterogeneity in symptom presentation seen in

TABLE 1.3   Clinical Manifestations of HIV Infection in Children

Failure to thrive (decreased weight gain and growth)
Fever
Gastrointestinal dysfunction (recurrent diarrhea)
Generalized lymphadenopathy
Hepato-splenomegaly
Persistent and severe oral candidiasis
Bacterial infections (e.g., otitis media, pneumonia)
Parotid enlargement
Lymphocystic interstitial pneumonia (LIP)
Multiple organ system involvement
Opportunistic infections (e.g., PCP)
Neurologic abnormalities (e.g., developmental delay, cognitive deficits,
  microcephaly)

infants and young children. Indeed, the range of clinical abnormalities in HIV-infected children extends from no detectable abnormalities to widespread systemic involvement. The age of onset, number, severity, and duration of symptoms listed in Table 1.3 can and does vary significantly from child to child. Failure to thrive, fever, gastrointestinal dysfunction (e.g., recurrent diarrhea), generalized lymphadenopathy, hepato-splenomegaly, and persistent and severe oral candidiasis or thrush are the most common symptoms, occurring in approximately one half of HIV-infected children (Ammann, 1990; Grossman, 1990; Rogers, 1989; Yolken, Hart, & Perman, 1991).

Unlike adults, children with HIV infection also have a much higher incidence (estimates range from 38% to 57%) of bacterial infections, including otitis media, sinusitis, pneumonia, sepsis, meningitis, and abscess of an internal organ. Urinary tract infection, skin and soft tissue infection, and gastroenteritis also have been commonly observed in HIV-infected children (Bernstein et al., 1985; Krasinski, Borkowsky, Bonk, Lawrence, & Chandwani, 1988). In response to the increased rate of bacterial infection in children, the 1987 CDC revision of the AIDS case definition included multiple or recurrent bacterial infections as a new criterion for pediatric AIDS. (The case definition of AIDS in adults does not include multiple or recurrent bacterial infections as a criterion.) Although the precise role of bacterial infection in the progression of HIV is not clear, children with HIV who develop serious bacterial infection are at increased risk of death (Pelton & Klein, 1991).

Additional clinical features not typically seen in adults but considered relatively common in children are parotid enlargement and lymphoid interstitial pneumonitis (LIP). Parotid enlargement occurs in approximately 15% of children, is typically bilateral and painless, and may persist for several months (Grossman, 1990). Lymphoid interstitial pneumonitis (or pulmonary lymphoid hyperplasia) occurs in about 40% of children, has an insidious onset most frequently after one year of age, and usually precedes chronic lung disease (Grossman, 1990). LIP is not a frequent cause of death in children, however, and children with LIP generally have a better prognosis for long-term survival than children with other opportunistic infections (Scott et al., 1989).

Multiple organ systems also have been implicated, as cardiomyopathy, hepatic dysfunction, nephrosis, and dermatological manifestations have been described (Parks & Scott, 1987). Furthermore, although not initially considered principal symptoms of HIV in children, cytomegalovirus (CMV) infection and varicella (chicken pox) have important clinical ramifications. According to Bryson and Arvin (1991), CMV is a major cause of blindness and death in children with AIDS, and the severity and progression of varicella is exacerbated in HIV-infected children. Anemia also occurs in nearly all symptomatic children.

As with adults, several other opportunistic infections have been observed in HIV-infected children. The most common and most life-threatening opportunistic infection in children is *Pneumocystis carinii* pneumonia (PCP), which is characterized by tachypnea (rapid breathing), dyspnea (shortness of breath), fever, and cough. Hughes (1991), in his review of PCP in children, reported that about 50% of children with AIDS can be expected to have PCP and that children younger than 1 year of age are significantly more vulnerable (72%) than older children (38%). Kaposi's sarcoma and primary B-cell lymphoma also have been reported in children, but their occurrence is far less frequent in children than in adults (Grossman, 1990).

Neurologic disease is another common clinical finding during the course of HIV infection. Indeed, HIV infection appears to have its most profound effect on the developing brain (Rosenberg & Fauci, 1991), although the neurological symptomatology in children with HIV infection is highly variable. Belman and her colleagues (Belman et al., 1985, 1988), in the largest longitudinal study of neurological complications in children with HIV infection yet reported, found that approximately 50% to 60% of children have neurologic abnormalities by the time they become symptomatic, whereas 85% to 90% demonstrate clear neurologic findings as the disorder progresses. The most frequent neurological manifestations of HIV infection in children include cognitive deficits, developmental abnormalities, acquired microcephaly, and progressive bilateral corticospinal tract signs.

As noted, neurological complications vary considerably in children, regardless of the mode of HIV transmission. Neurologic abnormalities may be secondary to opportunistic disease, central nervous system (CNS) tumors, and vascular problems, or they may occur in the absence of any opportunistic infection. Furthermore, progression of neurologic disease may be slow, intermittent, or rapid and may include developmental delay, loss of previously attained developmental milestones, attentional deficits, and intellectual deterioration. Developmental disabilities tend to appear early in the disease process, sometimes even preceding medical signs of infection, and tend to be more pervasive in children with more advanced disease. Microcephaly, seizures, and motor deficiencies manifested by paresis (partial paralysis), pathologic reflexes, ataxia, and gait disturbance also have been reported (Belman et al., 1988; Epstein, Sharer, & Goudsmit, 1988). Moreover, findings from computerized tomographic (CT) scans and magnetic resonance imaging (MRI) reveal cerebral atrophy, ventricular enlargement, calcifications, and attenuation of white matter (Brouwers, Belman, & Epstein, 1991).

Two additional points about the clinical manifestations of HIV infection in children are noteworthy. First, children who have acquired HIV infection via blood transfusion appear to follow a slightly different course than children who have been vertically infected (CDC, 1984). Although three fourths of children with hemophilia in the United States are now seropositive because of transfusions of widely infected concentrates of Factors VIII and IX received between 1979 and 1985, many of these children remain asymptomatic (Grossman, 1990). Thus there is some evidence that the incubation period is longer for children with parenterally transmitted HIV infection (Eyster, 1991). The clinical course and prognosis following the onset of AIDS symptoms, however, are comparable to those of young children who have acquired HIV infection via vertical transmission. Second, because HIV in children is a recent phenomenon, caution should be exercised in interpreting data describing the clinical course of HIV infection. Because of the relatively small number of infected children and the large proportion of children who remain asymptomatic, researchers examining the course of HIV infection have given necessarily greater attention to children with shorter asymptomatic periods (Rosenberg & Fauci, 1991).

Cofactors

Cofactors are those additional variables that predispose individuals to HIV infection (transmission cofactors) and those that affect the progression from HIV infection to symptom onset, AIDS, and death (progression cofactors). Cofactors currently under investigation in the adult AIDS literature include both biological (e.g., genetic predisposition to disease expression, presence of latent viral infections) and sociocultural (e.g., risk behavior, general health status) variables.

Factors affecting the probability of mother-to-infant transmission have not been elucidated. Although most studies report a vertical transmission rate of 25% to 40% (e.g., Douard et al., 1989; Falloon, Eddy, Wiener, & Pizzo, 1989), it is presently not known what proportion of this transmission occurs in utero, during labor and delivery, or postnatally during breast feeding (Rogers, 1989). Indeed, delivery mode and breast feeding have not been consistent predictors of vertical transmission of HIV (European Collaborative Study, 1988; Falloon et al., 1989; Italian Multicentre Study, 1988). Other factors considered important in explaining the differential mother-to-infant transmission rate include mother's history of viral infection, stage of HIV infection, lymphocyte levels, presence of neutralizing antibodies, and continued exposure to HIV during pregnancy; nature and degree of maternal drug use; and maternal and fetal infections other than HIV (Haverkos & Smeriglio, 1991).

Although numerous investigators have examined the role of cofactors in adult AIDS (Haverkos, 1987; Haverkos & Smeriglio, 1991), systematic studies of factors affecting the progression of HIV infection in children are lacking. Variables such as race, maternal risk group, exposure to infectious agents, presence of other viruses (e.g., Epstein-Barr virus infection), and genetic composition (e.g., major histocompatibility complex) warrant immediate empirical consideration. The cofactor most often cited as playing a critical role in the progression of HIV infection and AIDS symptomatology is the child's age. Numerous researchers have found that HIV infection and AIDS progress more rapidly in children younger than 1 year of age than in older children (Krasinski et al., 1989; Scott et al., 1989). Precisely what accounts for faster disease progression in infants has not been determined, although the timing of vertical transmission and subsequent development of immune system functioning in the fetus have been implicated (Ammann, 1988).

Prognosis

Children with vertically acquired HIV infection generally have a poor prognosis, although length of survival seems to depend upon specific clinical manifestations. Parks and Scott (1987), for instance, described two clinical courses and their differential survival rates. The first group consisted of children whose primary clinical manifestation was an opportunistic infection. Characterized by early disease onset (i.e., within first year of life; mean age of diagnosis equal to 6 months) and rapid immune deterioration, this first group had a median survival of 5 months after diagnosis. The second group of children had LIP as its predominant clinical manifestation, and the diagnosis was not usually made until sometime during the second year of life (mean age at diagnosis equal to 14 months). Median survival time for this group was 19 months.

Overall, the median survival rate for children with AIDS is 9 to 10 months following diagnosis. The mortality rate among children under 12 months of age is considerably higher than that among children over 12 months of age (80% vs. 55%, respectively; Rogers et al., 1987). Some researchers have suggested that the onset of progressive neurological symptoms is associated with shorter survival time (Belman et al., 1985; Epstein et al., 1986, 1987). For example, children survive an average of 8 months following the first evidence of neurological disease, and prognosis is even worse if HIV infection originated within the nervous system (Epstein et al., 1987, 1988). The development of any opportunistic infection, particularly PCP, is associated with very poor prognosis in children, regardless of age of occurrence (Scott & Hutto, 1991).

Summary and Conclusions

Clearly, a basic understanding of the medical aspects of HIV infection and AIDS is necessary to comprehend more accurately the social and psychological sequelae experienced by infected children and their families. Unlike most other diseases of childhood, AIDS progresses rapidly and leads to death in all instances. It has the unique possibility of affecting and eventually killing more than one family member within the same time period. Children and adolescents with AIDS experience a vast range of acute and chronic illnesses that demand intensive outpatient and inpatient medical services. Indeed, frequent illness and hospitalization may represent insurmountable social and psychological challenges to those children and families whose coping resources are limited.

This chapter has reviewed virologic and immunologic features, clinical manifestations, diagnostic and classification issues, and prognostic indicators of HIV infection and AIDS in children. Several conclusions can be drawn from the literature reviewed. First, numerous advances have been made during the past decade in understanding HIV and AIDS in children. A clinical profile for children with HIV infection has been documented, although the spectrum and severity of clinical responses in children remains highly variable. Second, further elucidation of the etiology and pathogenesis of viral and bacterial infections in children is needed for the development of more efficacious prevention and treatment methods. Third, new diagnostic tools for the early detection of vertically acquired HIV infection hold promise for the future. Fourth, the relationship between probable cofactors and immunologic status in children needs further definition. Finally, despite rapid and impressive advances in knowledge and technology, the longevity rate among infants and children with AIDS remains painfully low.

TWO

Epidemiology

This chapter reviews the epidemiology of HIV infection and AIDS, with particular attention to their prevalence and incidence among children, adolescents, and childbearing women; geographic distribution in the United States and other nations; and factors affecting their acquisition and spread. Data gathered from AIDS surveillance reports, HIV seroprevalence surveys, laboratory or cohort studies of HIV transmission, and authoritative epidemiological reviews serve as the basis for this chapter. Given the rapid pace with which new AIDS information is disseminated, some might argue that an "AIDS update" is an oxymoron; nevertheless, an epidemiological review provides an important backdrop to understanding the state of the AIDS pandemic at the time of this volume.

Centers for Disease Control: AIDS Classification and Surveillance

The Centers for Disease Control's (CDC) case surveillance system for AIDS is frequently cited as providing the most comprehensive assessment of the AIDS pandemic. This system monitors the magnitude of morbidity and mortality attributable to HIV infection in the United States, monitors short- and long-term trends in the AIDS pandemic, alerts health professionals to important changes in trends, and makes future projections regarding morbidity and mortality (CDC, 1990a). Certainly, a better understanding of the extent, distribution, and rate of HIV infection permits more accurate projections regarding the future scope of the problem.

Originally published in 1982, the CDC surveillance definition of AIDS remains the primary mechanism for tracking AIDS cases in the United States. The surveillance definition of AIDS was revised in 1985 and again in 1987, reflecting newly acquired knowledge about the nature and progression of the disease. Interestingly, the 1985 revision resulted in the reclassification of less than 1% of previously reported cases and added only a few (less than 4% of the total) new cases, even fewer of whom were children. In contrast, in the year following the 1987 revision, there was a significant increase in the number of new pediatric AIDS cases as well as a rise in the number of defined AIDS cases among IV drug users, women, and minorities.

The current definition includes individuals who are symptomatic but for whom either AIDS has not been immunologically documented or other specific diseases have not been ruled out. Thus AIDS can be diagnosed presumptively based upon presenting symptomatology (Table 2.1). In the case of children less than 13 years of age, the AIDS surveillance definition is viewed as a subset of Class P-2 (see Table 1.2 in Chapter 1) in the CDC HIV classification system. In other words, children with failure to thrive and recurrent diarrhea (Subclass A), progressive neurological disease (Subclass B), lymphoid interstitial pneumonia (Subclass C), opportunistic infections (Subclass D-1), unexplained and recurrent serious bacterial infections (Subclass D-2), and various cancers (Subclass E-1) are also included in the AIDS surveillance definition.

Reporting of an infectious disease is a critical step in controlling and preventing its spread. To this end, health professionals are mandated to report individuals who meet the surveillance definition to their local or state AIDS surveillance unit (Chorba, Berkelman, Safford, Gibbs, & Hull, 1990). CDC is then contacted and provided with demographic information, including the patient's age, gender, ethnicity, geographic location, mode of HIV transmission, and the life-threatening illness at the time of AIDS diagnosis. The patient's death, without specifying its cause, is subsequently reported to CDC.

There are several factors that may affect prevalence and incidence estimates of HIV infection and AIDS. For example, like most

TABLE 2.1   A Partial Listing of Conditions Included in the AIDS Surveillance Definition (1987 revision)

Recurrent bacterial infections
Candidiasis (trachea, bronchi, lungs, esophagus)
Cytomegalovirus disease onset after 1 month of age
Cytomegalovirus retinitis (with loss of vision)
Cryptococcosis, extrapulmonary
Cryptosporidiosis, chronic intestinal
HIV encephalopathy
Chronic herpes simplex ulcer
Histoplasmosis, disseminated or extrapulmonary
Isosporiasis, chronic intestinal
Kaposi's sarcoma
Lymphoid interstitial pneumonitis
Lymphoma (brain, Burkitt's, immunoblastic sarcoma)
Pneumocystis carinii pneumonia
Progressive multifocal leukoencephalopathy
Toxoplasmosis of brain after 1 month of age
Wasting syndrome attributable to HIV

---

surveillance systems for infectious diseases, the AIDS surveillance system relies predominantly upon health professionals to report cases. Some have argued that the current system for reporting cases underestimates the scope of the AIDS pandemic. For example, researchers have found that data generated from health professionals is often incomplete and not representative of certain populations (Chorba et al., 1990). Although the public visibility and high priority of AIDS likely contributes to increased reporting of AIDS cases relative to other infectious diseases, it is apparent that many health professionals do not know the specific procedures for reporting cases in their state and sometimes choose not to report AIDS cases because of concerns regarding confidentiality (Chorba et al., 1990).

Another factor possibly contributing to an underestimate of the AIDS problem is that most of the diseases included in the surveillance definition are those seen predominantly in gay or bisexual men. Because gynecological disorders common to women with AIDS are not included in the surveillance definition, many cases in women are not being reported to CDC. Moreover, in some instances, individuals are not reported to CDC until the time of death, when it is revealed for the first time that the person was HIV infected. Although complete and accurate reporting of cases is not necessary for the surveillance system to be useful, underreporting certainly may have an adverse effect on current public health efforts to monitor the prevalence and incidence of HIV infection and AIDS.

Prevalence and Incidence
of HIV Infection and AIDS

Prevalence statistics show the extent of HIV infection and AIDS in the United States. Current estimates using back-calculation methods (CDC, 1990a) indicate that more than 1 million individuals in the United States are currently HIV infected, a 30% increase over the number of HIV infections reported through 1985. It is estimated that 111,000 to 122,000 people in this country currently live with AIDS.

Incidence pertains specifically to the growth of the AIDS pandemic at a given time. Although determining incidence is problematic for estimates of pediatric cases, the incidence of new HIV infections for adolescents can be obtained from groups of individuals who are routinely screened for HIV infection (e.g., Red Cross donors, military applicants) or from serial prevalence measurements (CDC, 1990c). Approximately 42,000 new cases of AIDS occurred in 1990, reflecting a 19% increase over the number of new cases reported in 1989 (CDC, 1991a). The annual rate of AIDS per 100,000 population increased from 13.6 in 1989 to 16.6 in 1990 (CDC, 1991a). In the following sections, prevalence and incidence estimates are reported for infants, children, adolescents, and women of childbearing age.

Infants, Children, and
Women of Childbearing Age

According to the CDC (1991a), in the United States through December 31, 1990, there were 2,620 reported cases of AIDS in children less than 13 years of age, representing slightly less than 2% of all individuals with AIDS. As noted in Figure 2.1, children less than 5 years of age constituted the largest percentage (67%) of reported AIDS cases among children and adolescents through 1990. Figure 2.2 presents the number of pediatric AIDS cases reported by year (1981-1990). Reported child and adolescent AIDS cases in 1990 rose by 19% over the 1989 level. Per 100,000 population, the incidence rate for

Less Than 5 Yrs Old
67%

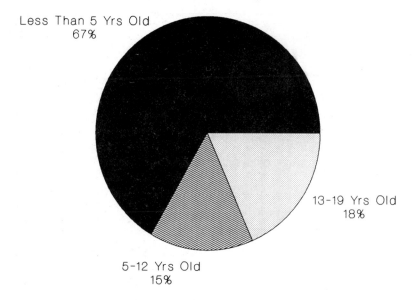

13-19 Yrs Old
18%

5-12 Yrs Old
15%

Figure 2.1. Percentage of Reported Pediatric AIDS Cases by Age Group
(through 1990)

AIDS is 2.8 for children less than 5 years of age; 0.5 for children 5 to
9 years old; and 0.4 for children and adolescents 10 to 19 years of
age. The cumulative (since 1982) incidence rate for vertically acquired
AIDS is approximately 4 per 100,000 children less than 13 years of
age.

Because vertical transmission now accounts for the largest percentage of AIDS cases among children, a more accurate assessment
of the scope of this pandemic in children might be achieved by examining AIDS among women of childbearing age. More than 15,000
(9% to 11%) cases of AIDS have been reported in women of childbearing age (CDC, 1990b). Between 1988 and 1989, the incidence rate
of AIDS among women increased by 29%, whereas the increase for
men was 18% during the same time period. Given the slower rate
of increase in AIDS cases among gay and bisexual men, women are
likely to account for a rapidly increasing percentage of AIDS cases
as the proportion of HIV infections via heterosexual contact continues its sharp incline (CDC, 1990f). Unfortunately, the dramatic rise
in the number of pediatric AIDS cases is directly proportional to the

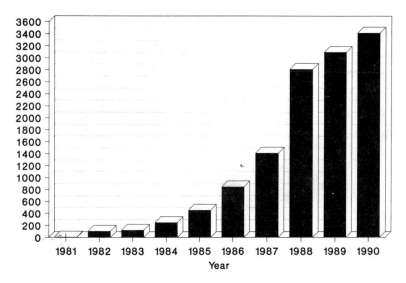

Figure 2.2. Number of Reported Pediatric AIDS Cases by Year (through 1989)
NOTE: 1990 data are provisional because the median delay in reporting cases to CDC exceeds 3 months.

growing number of women with HIV infection, now estimated at over 100,000.

Most states (44 states, the District of Columbia, and Puerto Rico) are participating in a national survey of childbearing women in which the prevalence of maternal HIV is determined through blind testing of newborn heel-stick blood samples taken routinely shortly after birth. The estimated national seroprevalence rate in 1989 was 0.15%, with a range of less than 0.10% for most states to 0.97% in the District of Columbia (Gwinn et al., 1990). Based upon this national survey, it is estimated that about 6,000 HIV-infected women are delivering infants each year, with a probable increase in subsequent years. Using a 30% rate of vertical transmission, Oxtoby (1991) estimated that each year, 1,600 to 1,800 children will acquire HIV infection via vertical transmission.

Despite an increase in AIDS cases being reported to CDC, several advocacy groups (e.g., ACT UP of New York City) have been spawned that have called attention to the increasing AIDS problem among women of childbearing age. They argue strongly that AIDS within this subgroup is underreported because the CDC surveillance definition does not recognize gynecological disorders common to women with AIDS, including vaginal thrush, tubo-ovarian abscesses, and pelvic inflammatory disease. Indeed, Chu, Buehler, and Berkelman (1990) recently found that 48% of women with known HIV infection or AIDS died of medical complications not presently recognized in the CDC surveillance definition. Moreover, as early as 1987, AIDS was the eighth leading cause of death among women 15 to 44 years of age in the United States (CDC, 1990b), and recent estimates indicate that it soon will become one of the top five causes of death in this subgroup (Chu et al., 1990). Indeed, in some geographical regions, this latter projection has already been surpassed: AIDS is now the leading cause of death among women 25 to 34 years of age in New York City (Drucker & Vermund, 1987). Clearly, as the incidence of HIV infection and AIDS (reported or not) rises in childbearing women, so too does the incidence of HIV and AIDS among children.

Adolescents

Despite recent efforts to recognize adolescents as a group at high risk for HIV infection (Hein, 1989; Manoff, Gayle, Mays, & Rogers, 1989), epidemiological information about this group is scant. Perhaps we know so little about adolescents because they constitute less than 1% (n = 629 through 1990) of individuals with AIDS and have drawn less public and empirical attention than younger children and adults. Indeed, the case can be made that AIDS among adolescents represents a significant health problem that has consistently been underestimated. More than 17,000 adolescents were thought to be HIV infected through 1987 (Stehr-Green, Bevers, & Berkelman, 1990), and current estimates of probable HIV infection among adolescents exceed 20,000. Blood testing conducted with adolescents attending clinics for sexually transmitted diseases, those applying to the military and the federal Job Corps program, and those seeking shelter in runaway facilities reveals an average HIV prevalence rate of about 0.50% (Gayle & D'Angelo, 1991).

A more accurate understanding of the AIDS epidemic among adolescents can be obtained by examining HIV infection and AIDS among young adults. Relative to young children, HIV infection during adolescence is characterized by a longer incubation period. Thus although HIV infection may occur during adolescence, symptoms may not become evident until early adulthood. Approximately 40% to 50% of the more than 6,000 AIDS cases reported since 1981 for young adults between 20 and 24 years of age can be traced to HIV infection during adolescence. An additional ominous sign regarding the AIDS epidemic among adolescents is the rising incidence of other sexually transmitted diseases among youths in the United States (Hein, 1989).

Three fourths of adolescent AIDS cases occur in those 17 to 19 years of age, and 75% of the total number of adolescents with AIDS are male (CDC, 1991a). Although the cumulative male to female ratio among adults is approximately 10:1, the male to female ratio for adolescents is 4:1. The male to female ratio is expected to drop over the next few years because of the dramatic increase in the number of adolescent female AIDS cases since 1987 and the decline in hemophilia-related AIDS cases among adolescent males.

Race/Ethnic Status

Distribution of AIDS cases by racial or ethnic group is disproportionate. Overall, African-Americans and Hispanic-Americans account for approximately 44% of all AIDS cases, but represent only 18% of the U.S. population (CDC, 1991a; Osmond, 1990a; Selik, Castro, & Pappaioanou, 1988). Moreover, the prevalence rate of HIV and the incidence of AIDS among children and women of childbearing age in the United States are highest among African-American and Hispanic-American populations (Gayle, Selik, & Chu, 1990; Selik et al., 1988). Indeed, the annual incidence of AIDS among children and women of childbearing age has increased steadily for most ethnic groups; however, the incidence of AIDS has remained persistently and disproportionately higher among African-American and Hispanic-American children and women than among those in other groups.

Figures 2.3 and 2.4 display the percentage distribution of AIDS cases among children and women of childbearing age, respectively, relative to the estimated population of these two groups (as well as whites) in the United States through 1989. Clearly, African-American and Hispanic-American children account for a disproportionate share of AIDS cases (78%) relative to their representation within the U.S. population (24%). Their cumulative AIDS incidence rates are

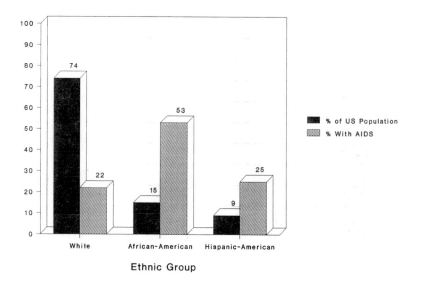

Figure 2.3. Percentage Distribution of Pediatric AIDS Cases Relative to the Estimated U.S. Child Population (1990)

21 and 13 times, respectively, higher than the incidence rates in white children.

Minority women of childbearing age similarly have a high incidence of AIDS relative to the proportion of the population they represent (75% vs. 21%). Seroprevalence studies involving female military applicants have found that African-American and Hispanic-American women have HIV infection rates four and eight times higher, respectively, than white female military applicants (Oxtoby, 1991). In a 1-year seroprevalence study conducted in the state of New York (Novick et al., 1989), 84% of the newborns with maternal HIV antibodies were African-American or Hispanic-American. Similarly, Mitchell and Heagarty (1991) reported recently that 85% of all vertically transmitted AIDS cases occur among ethnic minorities.

Not surprisingly, minorities also constitute a disproportionately high number of adolescent AIDS cases. Although African-American and Hispanic-American adolescents represent only 14% and 8%, respectively, of the population, they constitute 36% and 18%, respectively, of adolescent AIDS cases.

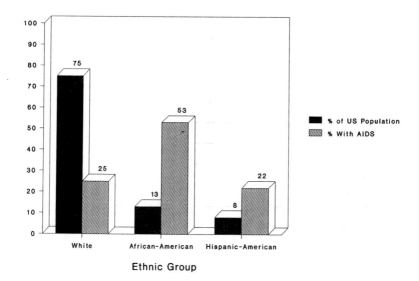

Figure 2.4. Percentage Distribution of AIDS Among Childbearing Women Relative to the Estimated U.S. Population (1990)

Geographic Distribution

Although pediatric AIDS cases have been reported in most states, New York, New Jersey, Florida, and the District of Columbia account for the vast majority of known cases. Vertical transmission secondary to IV drug use or sexual contact with an IV drug user is particularly prominent in New York, New Jersey, and the District of Columbia, with rapidly increasing numbers of such cases occurring in Florida. Nearly 70% of vertically acquired AIDS cases, but only about 18% of the general pediatric population, live in East Coast metropolitan areas (Oxtoby, 1991). Data from the national neonatal survey discussed previously suggest that New York and the District of Columbia will continue to be centers of HIV infection and AIDS among children and women of childbearing age. There is growing concern, though, that prevalence will increase among children and women in southeastern states, particularly Florida, because seroprevalence rates continue to rise in southern rural areas.

Adolescent AIDS cases have been reported in 41 states, the District of Columbia, and Puerto Rico, with the greatest concentration of cases (72%) having been diagnosed in large metropolitan areas, where only 42% of the total population resides (Gayle & D'Angelo, 1991). More than half of all adolescent AIDS cases have been reported from New York, Florida, California, Texas, New Jersey, and Puerto Rico.

Routes of HIV Transmission

Epidemiological studies consistently reveal that there are three primary modes of HIV transmission: sexual transmission (homosexual, bisexual, or heterosexual), parenteral transmission (transfusion of infected blood products, or injection with blood-contaminated needles/syringes), and vertical transmission (intrauterine, intrapartum, or postpartum). These modes of HIV transmission are discussed below as they pertain to infants, children, adolescents, and women of child-bearing age.

Vertical Transmission

As noted in Figure 2.5, vertical transmission accounts for approximately 84% of AIDS cases among children less than 13 years of age (CDC, 1991a). Vertical transmission will likely become the only route of pediatric HIV infection now that the risk of acquiring HIV infection from transfusion of contaminated blood or blood products has been virtually eliminated. Indeed, the prospects appear grim because the incidence of pediatric AIDS is directly proportional to the unsafe practices of IV drug users and their sexual partners, a rapidly growing transmission group among adults (Ammann, 1990). Fortunately, not every infected mother will transmit HIV to her offspring. As noted in Chapter 1, children born to infected mothers may possess maternal HIV antibodies for several months, thus making it difficult to determine the precise rate of actual HIV infection in newborns; however, the current rate of vertical transmission ranges from 25% to 40% (e.g., Blanche et al., 1989; European Collaborative Study, 1988; Hutto et al., 1991; Johnson et al., 1989).

Vertical transmission may occur in utero (intrauterine), during labor (intrapartum), or after birth (postpartum). The rates of infec-

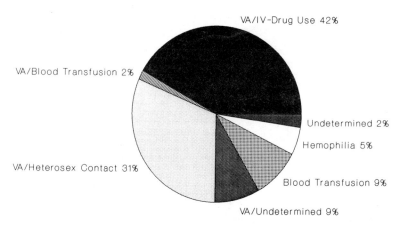

Figure 2.5. Percentage of Pediatric AIDS Cases by Patient Risk Group Through 1990 (children less than 13 years old)
NOTE: VA = Vertically Acquired AIDS

tion and degrees of risk associated with these specific transmission routes, however, have not been determined. Most medical authorities believe that vertical transmission occurs predominantly in utero, though the precise timing of infection during pregnancy has not been determined. Transplacental HIV transmission was initially described in 1985 when it was discovered postmortem that a newborn delivered via cesarean section possessed HIV-infected lymphoid cells (Lapointe, Michaud, Pekovic, Chausseau, & Dupuy, 1985). Subsequently, researchers have found evidence of in-utero infection by isolating HIV in aborted fetuses (Sprecher, Soumenkoff, Puissant, & Degueldre, 1986), from neonatal-cord blood lymphocytes (Di Maria et al., 1986), and by polymerase chain reaction tests (see Chapter 1) within a few days after birth (Laure et al., 1988). Furthermore, there is evidence that the placenta may play a role in either preventing or permitting (or both) HIV transmission in utero (Hill, Bolton, & Carlson, 1987; Maury, Potts, & Rabson, 1989).

It also seems plausible that HIV is transmitted from mother to infant during the labor and delivery process. All infants are exposed to maternal blood during delivery, and infants born vaginally are also exposed to cervical secretions. As outlined by Andiman and Modlin (1991), there are several arguments supporting intrapartum infection, including the fact that other viruses (e.g., hepatitis B) have a very high rate of vertical transmission and the finding that HIV is present in vaginal and cervical secretions in about 50% of HIV-infected women. Despite speculation regarding the role of labor and delivery in the transmission of HIV, however, conclusive empirical evidence regarding the occurrence of intrapartum transmission is lacking.

HIV reportedly has been detected in breast milk and colostrum (Friedland & Klein, 1987; Stiehm & Vink, 1991; Thiry et al., 1985; Vogt et al., 1986). Postpartum transmission of HIV via breast milk also has been reported, though the number of cases is quite small (Valdiserri, 1989; Weinbreck et al., 1988; Ziegler, Johnson, Cooper, & Gold, 1985) and the evidence inconclusive (Senturia, Ades, Peckham, & Giaquinto, 1987). In most instances, case reports describe mothers who acquired HIV after delivery and transmitted the virus to their infant via breast feeding. Several authors (e.g., Oxtoby, 1988; Ziegler, Stewart, Penny, Stuckey, & Good, 1988) have reported that the greatest risk of postpartum transmission may occur when the mother acquires HIV during the breast-feeding period. For instance, mothers acquiring HIV from blood transfusions after delivery may have higher concentrations of the virus in their blood and other secretions relative to women with more long-standing HIV infection. Overall, although HIV infection via breast milk is rare and empirical data are lacking, the CDC continues to discourage breast feeding among HIV-infected women (CDC, 1985b).

There are several maternal factors that may affect the risk of vertical transmission, although they have not been empirically delineated. For example, advanced maternal HIV symptomatology, preterm delivery, increased maternal age, and various immunologic features have been associated with increased risk of vertical transmission (Andiman & Modlin, 1991). Possible associations with the presence of sexually transmitted diseases other than HIV are currently under investigation. Thus the clinical course of HIV infection during gestation and symptomatology unrelated to HIV may be important variables in elucidating the rate of vertical transmission.

Modes of Transmission Among Adolescents

Adolescents acquire HIV and AIDS in the same ways that adults do: IV drug use, male homosexual/bisexual contact, male homosexual/bisexual contact with an IV drug user, heterosexual contact,

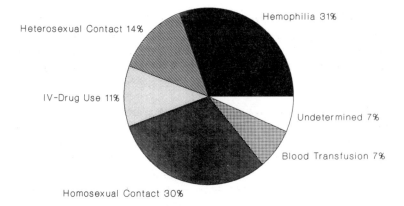

Figure 2.6. Percentage of Adolescent AIDS Cases by Patient Risk Group (through 1990)

blood transfusion, and blood products secondary to hemophilia or coagulation disorders. Figure 2.6 illustrates the distribution of adolescent AIDS cases by risk category. Like adults, behavioral factors (i.e., IV drug use, sexual contact) account for more than half (55%) of the reported cases of HIV infection among adolescents. Transfusion of blood products accounts for about 38% of known adolescent AIDS cases.

Modes of HIV transmission among adolescents vary considerably according to age, gender, and race. For instance, the incidence of HIV infection because of transfusions of blood or blood products is highest among young adolescents aged 13 to 14 years and lowest among adolescents aged 17 to 19 years. Conversely, the percentage of adolescent HIV infection attributable to IV drug use or sexual contact with an infected partner ranges from 9% for young adolescents to approximately 70% for those 17 to 19 years old.

Adolescent males and females appear to have distinctly different patterns of HIV transmission. For adolescent males, homosexual or bisexual contact accounts for the greatest percentage of known AIDS cases (43%), followed by hemophilia or coagulation disorders (38%) and IV drug use (7%). Because HIV infection among people with hemophilia and other coagulation disorders is seen predominantly in young adolescent males (87%), and because the rate of HIV infection through transfusions continues to decline, the percentage of adolescent AIDS cases accounted for by homosexual or bisexual activity and IV drug use will likely increase significantly. Behavior-related exposure accounts for an even greater percentage of AIDS cases among adolescent females: heterosexual contact (44%) and IV drug use (28%) account for the largest percentage of AIDS cases among this subgroup.

Overall, the outlook for attenuating the rising trend of HIV infection among adolescents is dismal. On a positive note, more effective methods for heat treatment of clotting factors and mandatory nationwide screening of blood donors have resulted in a negligible risk (less than 1%) of new HIV infection among adolescents with hemophilia and among those receiving blood transfusions (Eyster, 1991), although adolescents infected prior to such changes represent a highly infectious population. Furthermore, from 1989 to 1990 there was a 12% decrease in the number of adolescent AIDS cases secondary to homosexual or bisexual activity.

Overby, Lo, and Litt (1989), however, found that despite adequate knowledge about safe sexual practices, only one in nine male adolescents with hemophilia used condoms during sexual intercourse. Additionally, adolescent sexual activity is high, the age at first intercourse is declining, and the number of sexual partners is increasing (CDC, 1991b; O'Reilly & Aral, 1985); the number who consistently use contraceptive devices remains relatively low (Kegeles, Adler, & Irwin, 1988; O'Reilly & Aral, 1985); receptive anal intercourse, a particularly high-risk factor for HIV transmission, is now a common practice among minority adolescent females as a means of avoiding pregnancy (Jaffe, Seehaus, Wagner, & Leadbetter, 1988); and increased drug use among adolescents may lead to a concomitant increase in high-risk sexual behavior (Fullilove, Fullilove, Bowser, & Gross, 1990). Adolescent sexual behavior and drug use as they relate to the AIDS crisis are discussed further in Chapters 4 and 5, respectively.

Women of Childbearing Age:
IV Drug Use and Heterosexual Contact

The sharing of needles during parenteral use of drugs is the predominant mode of HIV transmission for women of childbearing age (52%), followed by heterosexual contact with an infected partner (32%) and blood transfusions (11%; CDC, 1990c). The remaining 5% are classified as "undetermined" because the specific risk factors are presently unknown. Perhaps the most significant trend within this population is the hundredfold increase of heterosexually transmitted HIV within the last five years (Guinan & Hardy, 1987). Of even greater concern is the finding that as many as half of the women infected via sexual contact do not recognize that their partner is infected or at increased risk (Landesman, Minkoff, Hollman, McCalla, & Sijn, 1987).

Other Hypothesized Routes of HIV Transmission

Although HIV has been isolated from saliva, tears, and urine, there is no evidence that HIV can be transmitted through these bodily fluids (Lifson, 1988). Likewise, no epidemiological evidence for casual transmission of HIV has been found (Fischl et al., 1987; Friedland et al., 1986), and several studies have shown no evidence of HIV transmission through insects (e.g., Castro et al., 1988; Srinivasan, York, & Bohan, 1987). Rare cases of possible HIV transmission during an invasive dental procedure (CDC, 1990e, 1991c), following organ transplantation (CDC, 1987d), and after artificial insemination (CDC, 1990d; Stewart et al., 1985) have been reported.

Epidemiology of HIV Infection and AIDS in Other Nations

Although this review of the AIDS pandemic has focused primarily on children and adolescents residing in the United States, HIV infection and AIDS have no geographical boundaries. Indeed, AIDS cases have been reported from 152 countries around the world. Children and women of childbearing age in regions of Africa and the Caribbean have been most affected by the HIV pandemic. In contrast with developed countries, where pediatric AIDS represents only about 2% of all AIDS cases, in many developing countries pediatric AIDS constitutes 15% to 20% of the total reported cases (Piot, Plummer, Mhalu, Chin, & Mann, 1988). Even these figures may underrepresent the scope of the pediatric AIDS problem, because a large number of children in developing countries die from common childhood diseases (e.g., failure to thrive, chronic diarrhea, recurrent respiratory infections) before they begin to manifest AIDS symptomatology.

Current data estimate that more than 100,000 infants have been infected with HIV in parts of Africa, and approximately 250,000 infants are expected to be vertically infected by 1992 (Quinn, Ruff, & Halsey, 1991). HIV seroprevalence rates among pregnant women in Africa are estimated to be approximately 20% to 30% (Rwandan HIV Seroprevalence Study Group, 1989), and the vertical transmission rate in one African hospital was 73% (contrasted with 25% to 35% in the United States; Andiman & Modlin, 1991). Also, because the distribution of HIV infection and AIDS cases among males and females is equal in most developing countries, and because heterosexual contact is the primary cause of HIV infection (more than 80% of cases in Africa), the percentage of pediatric AIDS cases is expected to rise even higher during the next decade. Blood transfusions continue to be a significant problem in many developing regions (there is a 2% to 18% infection rate among donors in Africa) because economic and technical limitations have precluded complete implementation of appropriate blood screening methods. HIV exposure among older adolescents and young adults ranges from 25% to 35% (Biggar, 1986; Osmond, 1990b).

Although most regions of Asia and the Pacific have not reported a large number of AIDS cases, there has been a sharp increase in HIV infection because of IV drug use and prostitution in Thailand (Oxtoby, 1991). In Europe, more than 70% of pediatric AIDS cases are attributable to vertical transmission; France, Italy, and Spain have the highest number of pediatric AIDS cases caused by vertical transmission. Romania and the republics of the former Soviet Union also have experienced recent outbreaks of HIV in children.

HIV and AIDS symptomatology among children in developing nations closely resembles that seen in children in developed countries. Symptoms include failure to thrive, recurrent fever, chronic diarrhea, generalized lymphadenopathy, and recurrent bacterial infections. There are some differences, however, in the clinical course of AIDS among children in developing countries. For example, severe protein-energy malnutrition and nontyphoid salmonella occur more frequently among children from developing countries than among children in the United States and parts of Europe. Disease progression is also more rapid among children in developing regions. HIV-infected children in Africa do more poorly in the first 2 years of life; about 50% die by age 24 months, compared to 20% in the United States and some European countries (Ryder et al., 1989). The geographical discrepancy in how quickly the disease progresses has been attributed to increased infectious exposures, malnutrition, illness in the infant's primary caretaker, lack of specific therapies, poor availability of timely medical care for management of bacterial infections, and differences in virus strains in developing regions (Oxtoby, 1991; Quinn et al., 1991).

Developing countries also differ from the developed world in their diagnostic methods and case definition. Many standard HIV diagnostic tools (e.g., ELISA, PCR) used in developed regions are not yet being used routinely in developing countries. The costs of these tests are astronomically high, and many countries lack the laboratory personnel, equipment, and electrical power necessary to coordinate such testing efficiently. Similarly, medical tests and equipment necessary to detect secondary infections and malignancies commonly associated with HIV infection and AIDS often are either unavailable or unattainable. Because of the lack of appropriate or accurate diagnostic techniques, many developing regions use a case definition that is based entirely on clinical findings. Unfortunately, many of the clinical findings in these case definitions are nonspecific and are seen commonly among children without HIV infection. Case definitions in developing countries also tend to emphasize symptoms associated with wasting syndrome while ignoring pulmonary manifestations, which are the initial presenting symptom of many HIV-infected children in the United States and Europe (Berkley, Okware, & Naamara, 1989). Insufficient viral detection methods and restricted case definitions pose similar problems for HIV-2, a retrovirus distinct from HIV-1 that has been isolated in individuals in West Africa.

Summary and Conclusions

The incidence of HIV infection and AIDS among infants, children, adolescents, and childbearing women has risen sharply in recent years, and there is no epidemiological evidence that this trend will ease any time soon. For instance, the CDC (1990b) projects the cumulative total of U.S. AIDS cases resulting from vertical transmission to reach 14,000 by the end of 1993.

African-Americans and Hispanic-Americans are disproportionately affected by AIDS in the United States. Surveillance data clearly indicate that IV drug use and sex with an IV drug user are the principal routes of HIV transmission among African-American and Hispanic-American adolescents and childbearing women. Education and prevention efforts must focus on specific drug-related issues as well as the diverse cultural factors represented within these particular ethnic groups.

A revision of current AIDS surveillance methods is needed to account more accurately for the growing number of AIDS cases and to reflect the true picture of HIV morbidity in children, adolescents, and childbearing women. Unfortunately, although the reported incidence of AIDS is tragically high, it appears that the scope of the HIV pandemic has been underestimated significantly. Infected children who are asymptomatic or whose symptomatology is not otherwise characteristic of advanced disease typically are not reported for surveillance purposes. Similarly, the omission of gynecological disorders from the AIDS surveillance definition leads to an underreporting of AIDS cases among women of childbearing age.

Elucidation of epidemiological trends also must continue. Specifically, regional and national studies examining trends in HIV transmission categories among adolescents and childbearing women are especially important. Further clarification regarding the timing and specific mechanisms of vertical transmission and a clear delineation of the maternal factors associated with this transmission route are also warranted.

THREE

Knowledge and Attitudes

The empirical literature concerning youths' knowledge about and attitudes toward AIDS is reviewed in this chapter. *Knowledge* refers to factual information about the disease, and *attitudes* refer to more emotionally laden responses, such as fear, worry, and concern about AIDS and about persons with AIDS. As discussed in Chapter 6, an accurate understanding of children's and adolescents' knowledge and attitudes concerning AIDS is necessary for the design of efficacious education and prevention efforts. In light of the almost complete absence of information regarding children's knowledge about and attitudes toward AIDS (see DeLoye, Henggeler, & Daniels, 1992), however, this review focuses on adolescents and college students. Before youths' knowledge and attitudes concerning AIDS are reviewed, several methodological considerations evident in this literature will be addressed.

Methodological Considerations

Cook and Campbell (1979) have noted four broad aspects of research methodology that threaten the integrity of findings: construct validity, internal validity, external validity, and statistical conclusion validity. As described below, there are many significant methodological limitations in the literature examining youths' knowledge and attitudes regarding AIDS. It should be emphasized, however, that such limitations are typical in newly emerging areas of research.

Construct Validity

Construct validity pertains to the capacity of research instruments to measure the constructs that they purport to measure. With few exceptions, the AIDS knowledge and attitude questionnaires used in this literature are not well validated. Although the items in these questionnaires usually have good face validity, items often overlap, and their factor structures and internal consistencies rarely have been determined. Thus knowledge and attitude are treated as unidimensional constructs, when in fact they probably are multidimensional. Moreover, single items often are used to measure key constructs despite that fact that one-item measures are notoriously unreliable. Exceptions to this tendency are a recently developed 54-item AIDS Attitude Scale (Shrum, Turner, & Bruce, 1989) that includes factors that tap moral issues, social welfare issues, and concerns regarding proximity with people with AIDS; and a separate 15-item AIDS Attitude Scale (Bliwise, Grade, Irish, & Ficarrotto, 1991) that includes factors that assess health care workers' fear of contagion, negative emotions, and professional resistance.

Forced-choice response formats represent another significant problem with the scales used in this literature. Leading questions often are included (e.g., "Have you changed your sexual behavior since learning of AIDS?"), and respondents typically are given the choice of three responses (e.g., true, false, don't know). In such cases, interpretations of results do not weigh the probability of selecting a particular response by chance. For example, what does it mean when 50% of respondents answer "true" when asked to agree or disagree with the statement, "You can get AIDS by kissing someone with the disease"? Do 50% of the respondents actually believe this, or has a percentage of the respondents just guessed? It seems likely that open-ended questions will elicit different and possibly more accurate information concerning youths' knowledge of and attitudes toward AIDS (see, e.g., Brown, Nassau, & Levy, 1990). In any case, the continued use of poorly validated research instruments greatly threatens the internal validity of findings.

Internal Validity

Several threats to internal validity (i.e., establishing the true association among variables) are pervasive in the knowledge and attitudes literature. First, as noted previously, many of the measurement instruments are not well validated. Second, when attitudes toward AIDS are assessed, comparisons needed to provide a frame of reference for the results rarely are included. For example, it is difficult to interpret the significance of a finding that "50% of youths fear AIDS" in the absence of similar data regarding other childhood fears. Is the fear of AIDS more frequent or qualitatively greater than the fear of cancer or the fear of one's parents arguing? Third, it is similarly difficult to judge the extent of a sample's knowledge about AIDS when comparison groups are not included in the study.

Fourth, investigators have evaluated respondents' attitudes toward AIDS without first determining what the respondents knew about AIDS. This is especially problematic for elementary-school-age children. Fifth, knowledge and attitudes are changing rapidly, and empirical relationships that might be valid at one point in time may not be valid at a later date. Sixth, minimal attention has been devoted to third-variable alternative interpretations (e.g., psychosocial characteristics of respondents and their families) that may weaken observed associations among variables. For example, although it may be tempting to draw a causal inference from an observed association between knowing that condom use reduces risk of AIDS and reported use of condoms, there are many third variables that might account for this relationship (e.g., intelligence and social competence may each be associated with knowledge and condom use). Seventh, Bliwise et al. (1991) have shown that health care professionals' attitudes toward AIDS are significantly associated with social desirability. There is no apparent reason to believe that the attitudes of youths would not show similar social-desirability effects. Hence, consistent with the suggestions of Bliwise and her colleagues, future investigators should consider the role of social desirability in their results.

External Validity

External validity refers to the generalizability of findings. It is determined largely by the characteristics and representativeness of the sample. In the absence of major funding, it is difficult to accrue other than a convenience sample. Even in those few cases when a probability sample has been assessed—through random-digit dialing, for example (Strunin & Hingson, 1987)—important segments of the population often are excluded (e.g., incarcerated youths, homeless youths, families without phones). Nevertheless, most investigators are well aware of the limitations presented by their samples and carefully describe these limitations. One aspect of external validity, however, often has been ignored: Relatively few investigators have examined the effects of moderating variables such as gender, ethnicity, and age. Such evaluations would provide important information regarding the generalizability of the findings.

Statistical Conclusion Validity

Here, the primary threats to the integrity of findings are statistical power and inflation of Type I error. In general, studies of knowledge and attitudes regarding AIDS have included large samples; consequently, statistical power is usually high. On the other hand, Type I error often is inflated by the use of numerous univariate statistical tests without modifying alpha (e.g., with the Bonferonni correction) and by the failure to use multivariate analyses.

In summary, the literature regarding knowledge about and attitudes toward AIDS includes many significant methodological limitations. Nevertheless, many of the studies have been heuristic and have made substantive contributions. The relatively well-designed studies are reviewed more extensively in the subsequent sections.

Adolescents' Knowledge and Misconceptions About AIDS

Early investigations indicated that adolescents had limited knowledge about AIDS and held numerous misconceptions. Price, Desmond, and Kukulka (1985) assessed a convenience sample of 250 high school students in the Midwest using a knowledge questionnaire with a three-choice response format (true, false, don't know). Although 90% of the students knew that homosexuals were at risk for AIDS, only 40% indicated that drug users were at risk. Moreover,

50% did not know that Orientals were not at increased risk. In a second early study (N = 1,326; DiClemente, Zorn, & Temoshok, 1986), the authors concluded that San Francisco high school students' knowledge was uneven. Using a knowledge questionnaire with a three-choice format, the investigators found that 92% of the students knew that sexual intercourse was one mode of contracting AIDS, but only 60% knew that condom use lowered the risk, and only 75% knew that AIDS could not be contracted by shaking hands.

Studies conducted more recently have shown that adolescents have relatively high levels of knowledge about AIDS. With a convenience sample of 189 adolescents attending AIDS seminars, Manning and Balson (1989) found that more than 90% of the youths knew that AIDS was transmitted through sexual relations, IV drug use, and blood contact; 91% knew that condom use lowered the risk of contracting AIDS. Similar results were obtained by Reid (1988) in a sample of adolescents in Fife, Great Britain. Likewise, three studies with adolescent women attending family-planning clinics found that the respondents had relatively high levels of knowledge about AIDS (Beaman & Strader, 1989; Seltzer, Rabin, & Benjamin, 1989; Weisman et al., 1989). The results of these latter studies are noteworthy for several reasons. First, the women in these samples either had a sexually transmitted disease (STD; Beaman & Strader, 1989) or were at high risk for STDs and, as such, were at risk for AIDS. Second, the samples included high percentages of minority and economically disadvantaged participants. Third, Seltzer et al. (1989) assessed the youths' knowledge with an open-ended interview method, which is much more demanding on the respondents than a questionnaire with a true-false format.

Hingson and his colleagues have presented the most convincing evidence of the increased knowledge about AIDS among adolescents (Hingson, Strunin, & Berlin, 1990). They contrasted the results from two independent random-digit-dialing surveys conducted statewide in Massachusetts in 1986 (N = 860; Strunin & Hingson, 1987) and 1988 (N = 1,762; Hingson et al., 1990). The percentage of correct responses increased from 91% to 99% for knowing that AIDS can be transmitted both through heterosexual relations and by injecting drugs. In addition, the percentage of incorrect responses decreased from 38% to 11% for indicating the sharing of eating utensils as a transmission route and from 58% to 25% for agreeing that kissing is a transmission route. As these latter figures indicate, misconceptions are still held by numerous youths. Nevertheless, it appears that educational efforts and/or media exposure generally have been successful at increasing adolescents' knowledge about AIDS.

College Students' Knowledge and Misconceptions

Several groups of investigators, using convenience samples, have assessed college students' knowledge and misconceptions about AIDS (Fisher & Misovich, 1990; Goodwin & Roscoe, 1988; Gottlieb, Vacalis, Palmer, & Conlon, 1988; Katzman, Mulholland, & Sutherland, 1988; Manning, Barenberg, Gallese, & Rice, 1989; McDermott, Hawkins, Moore, & Cittadino, 1987). In general, these investigators have concluded that college students have relatively high levels of knowledge about AIDS, although some misconceptions were evident. For example, in a large-scale survey of college students across 17 diverse colleges and universities, DiClemente, Forrest, Mickler et al. (1990) found that 97% of respondents knew that AIDS can be transmitted through vaginal intercourse and 93% knew that AIDS can be transmitted by someone who is infected but does not have any symptoms of the disease. On the other hand, 31% of the college students thought that AIDS could be transmitted by kissing, and 4% thought that one could get AIDS from swimming pools. DiClemente and his colleagues concluded that knowledge and misconceptions were two conceptually distinct domains of information and that providing students with accurate information will not necessarily dispel misconceptions. Moreover, as discussed later in this chapter, misconceptions about transmission routes are linked with the anxiety and fear associated with AIDS.

Youths' Knowledge and Misconceptions Relative to the General Public

Investigators of knowledge about AIDS usually have concluded that the respondents in their samples had "high" or perhaps "low" levels of knowledge. Rarely, however, has more than one type of respondent (e.g., high school students, clinic patients) been surveyed in a particular study. Without an appropriate referent, it seems difficult to discern whether a particular group of respondents has a high or low level of knowledge, as *high* and *low* are relative terms. For example, Richwald, Sekler, Kitimbo, and Friedland (1989) surveyed students pursuing graduate degrees in public health and concluded that the findings "raise serious concern about the level of knowledge about HIV and AIDS" (p. 93). Although such a conclusion might have been warranted, it is also possible that these students had more knowledge than did other types of health care professionals.

In the preceding review, we concluded that youths generally have high levels of knowledge about AIDS. In support of this conclusion, Table 3.1 presents several results from the National Health Interview Survey (NHIS) conducted from August through December in 1987 (Dawson, 1988). The NHIS is a continuous household interview survey designed to represent the entire civilian, noninstitutionalized adult population of the United States. This survey included a 6-point response in which two choices ("very unlikely" and "definitely not possible") were correct for items assessing misconceptions (e.g., whether AIDS could be transmitted through kissing, toilet seats, or sharing eating utensils), and one choice ("very likely") was correct for items assessing knowledge (e.g., whether AIDS could be transmitted through heterosexual relations or sharing needles). As a comparison, the results from large-scale surveys of high school students in early 1988 (Hingson et al., 1990) and college students from March through November of 1987 (DiClemente et al, 1990) also are presented. Although sampling (e.g., random vs. convenience) and measurement (e.g, 3-point vs. 6-point response format) issues must be weighed when comparing the results of these studies, the data support the contention that, in general, youths have relatively high levels of knowledge about AIDS.

Moderators of Youths' Knowledge and Misconceptions

As knowledge about AIDS becomes more widespread, it may be efficacious to target additional educational efforts at those individuals who are likely to have knowledge deficits. Within the general adult population, there is strong evidence that knowledge is associated with age, ethnicity, and education, but not with gender (Dawson, 1988; Dawson & Hardy, 1989). Several of the studies discussed previously examined moderating factors regarding adolescents' knowledge. Price et al. (1985) found that boys had greater knowledge than girls on 40% of the items in their questionnaire; the authors suggested

TABLE 3.1 Proportions of Correct Responses From Surveys of the General
Public, High School Students, and College Students

Can you get AIDS from:	General Public[a] (N = 17,000)	High School Students[b] (N = 1,762)	College Students[c] (N = 1,127)
sharing eating utensils?	33	89	61
kissing on the mouth?	14	75	52
toilet seat?	46	95	–
heterosexual sex?	92	99	97
sharing needles?	92	99	98

[a]Dawson (1988).
[b]Hingson et al. (1990).
[c]DiClemente et al. (1990).

that this finding reflected the greater interest of boys in this health problem. Manning and Balson (1989) evaluated the influence of adolescent age on knowledge and found no effects. In studies of college students, several investigators found no relationship between knowledge and gender (Manning et al., 1989; McDermott et al., 1987; Strader & Beaman, 1989). In addition, Manning et al. (1989) found that knowledge was not associated with students' religion, and McDermott et al. (1987) found that knowledge was not related to students' sexual orientation (e.g., heterosexual vs. homosexual/bisexual). In light of the scant information regarding moderating effects on knowledge and the minimal cost of evaluating such data (i.e., moderating variables are collected routinely during assessment sessions), we recommend that future investigators include such subgroup analyses. Moreover, little is known about the knowledge of youths who are on the fringes of society (e.g., the homeless, dropouts, incarcerated offenders) and who are at increased risk for contracting the disease.

Sources of AIDS-Related Information

There is consistent evidence that adolescents receive most of their information about AIDS from the popular media and that this information is perceived as credible. In a survey of seventh and eighth graders, Dolan, Corber, and Zacour (1990) found that television was the major source of information about AIDS for 69% of the youths, parents were the major source for 17%, friends for 5%, and health care professionals for 1%. Moreover, television was perceived as the most credible source by 39% of the students, followed by parents (28%), and health care professionals (19%). Likewise, Reid (1988) found that television was reported as a source of information about AIDS by 95% of their sample, and that 90% of these youths rated it as a credible source. In contrast, parents were reported as a source by 51% of the youths, with an 87% credibility rating. Health care professionals were rarely reported as sources of information, and they had relatively low credibility ratings when they were reported (except for "friends," the lowest credibility rating of all 12 possible sources was given to school nurses).

Similar findings regarding adolescents' sources of AIDS information were obtained by Price et al. (1985). Moreover, these authors evaluated whether AIDS knowledge was associated differentially with specific sources of information and found that respondents who reported the popular media as a source of their AIDS information had more knowledge about AIDS than those respondents who did not indicate popular media as an information source. No such differences were observed between groups of respondents who did versus those who did not report friends, family, or health care professionals as information sources. Similarly, Dolan et al. (1990) reported that adolescents who received AIDS information from their parents did not show increased knowledge compared with their counterparts who did not speak to their parents about AIDS.

The popular media have also been rated as the primary source of AIDS information by college students. McDermott et al. (1987) found that 93% of surveyed university students rated one of the popular media (television, newspapers, magazines, or radio) as their primary source of AIDS information. Friends were rated as the primary source by 3% of the students, and no respondent cited physicians as a primary source. Students' knowledge about AIDS was not associated with the type of popular media that was rated as the primary source. Although students obtain their information from the media, Manning et al. (1989) concluded that most college students would *prefer* to learn about AIDS from physicians rather than from the media, and that an AIDS patient was viewed as the second most desired source of information. The costs of such person-to-person educational efforts are probably prohibitive; nevertheless, the findings of Manning and his colleagues certainly have important implications for the design of educational efforts conducted through the media (at least for college students).

*Associations Between Knowledge
and Risk Behavior*

In cross-sectional studies, youths have reported that they changed their risk behaviors after learning about AIDS. Reports of such changes may lead investigators to conclude that knowledge about AIDS is associated with decreased risk behavior. Such a conclusion, however, is not supported in the literature. Aside from the problems with construct validity posed by these studies (e.g., leading questions that bias responses, low validity of assessing behavioral change with one static retrospective report), findings do not support a link between knowledge and behavior. For example, in their multisite study of college students, DiClemente and his colleagues (1990) found that many students reported that they decreased their risk behaviors after learning about AIDS. Changes in risk behaviors, however, were not associated with the level of the students' knowledge about AIDS. Moreover, Fisher and Misovich (1990) surveyed convenience samples of college students in three successive years and found that *increases* in knowledge about AIDS and in favorable attitudes toward condom use coincided with increases in the number of sexual partners and rates of unprotected sexual activity. Regarding high school students, Hingson et al. (1990) noted that the proportion of sexually active adolescents who reported adopting condom use because of AIDS increased from 2% in 1986 to 19% in 1988. Nevertheless, there were no differences in knowledge about AIDS among youths who adopted condom use to avoid AIDS versus those who did not. Thus, if youths have changed their behavior in response to AIDS, such changes seem unrelated to the extent of their knowledge about the disease.

Consistent with findings from the school-based surveys, clinic-based studies (Beaman & Strader, 1989; Hayes, Sharp, & Miner, 1989) that combined adolescents and adults in their samples have failed to find an association between knowledge and risk behavior. Weisman et al. (1989), on the other hand, found in their sample of adolescent clients at a family-planning clinic a marginally significant association between knowing that condom use reduces AIDS risk and reported condom use at last intercourse. Overall, however, it does not seem that the level of knowledge about AIDS is linked with risk behaviors. Consistent with the conclusions and recommendations of Becker and Joseph (1988), perhaps attitudes rather than information are associated more strongly with risk behaviors.

Attitudes Toward AIDS

Negative attitudes and fear about AIDS and toward persons with AIDS have been well documented in news reports ("AIDS Victim," 1985) and in public opinion polls (see, e.g., Singer, Rogers, & Corcoran, 1987). For example, based on interviews with a random sample of residents of a town in the Midwest, S. D. Johnson (1987) found that 61% of the respondents indicated that schools should not allow a child with AIDS to attend classes, and 49% indicated that there should be a law prohibiting people with AIDS from jobs that involve close contact with others.

Herek and Glunt's (1988) excellent overview of the sources of AIDS-related stigma is summarized here to provide a background for our subsequent review of the attitudes of adolescents, college students, and health care professionals about AIDS. These authors suggest that AIDS-related stigma and fear are associated with two distinct aspects of the disease: First, AIDS is a deadly illness; and second, it is associated with groups of persons who are already stigmatized.

Several aspects of AIDS as a deadly illness contribute to AIDS-related stigma and fear. First, it is an incurable, progressive, and transmissible disease that places others at risk. Second, AIDS is transmitted through voluntary behaviors; thus people infected with HIV are viewed as responsible for their plight. Third, the symptoms of AIDS-related illnesses are disfiguring. In addition, as Herek and Glunt noted, AIDS-related stigma is exacerbated by the association of the disease with marginalized groups such as homosexuals, illegal drug users, and minorities. Thus the public perceptions of AIDS are inextricably linked with two almost universal fears: death and outsiders.

Attitudes of Children and Adolescents

Investigators uniformly have concluded from school-based studies that a high percentage of youths is worried and fearful about AIDS, and clinical cases of AIDS-related anxiety disorders have been documented (e.g., Lewin & Williams, 1988). The percentage of youths reporting that they were afraid of getting AIDS has been estimated at 79% (DiClemente et al., 1986), 45% (Dolan et al., 1990), and 66% (King & Gullone, 1990); and 75% of adolescents in one study ranked AIDS as one of their three greatest fears (Brown & Fritz, 1988). Moreover, Hingson et al. (1990) found in their Massachusetts survey that the percentage of youths who were worried about AIDS increased from 46% in 1986 to 74% in 1988. As is usually the case with anxieties during adolescence, higher percentages of girls than boys have reported fear of AIDS (Dolan et al., 1990; King & Gullone, 1990). In addition, responses to several questionnaire items provide good examples of the extent of youths' fear of AIDS. Fifty-one percent of respondents in one study answered "true" to "I'd rather get any other disease than AIDS" (DiClemente et al., 1986); 28% of respondents in another would want to avoid a friend who had AIDS, and 32% would not allow students with AIDS to attend regular classes (Dolan et al., 1990). Moreover, age trends in attitudes toward AIDS have been observed (Brown et al., 1990), with 5th graders more concerned about the lethality of AIDS and 10th graders more concerned with their perceived helplessness. In summary, as one might expect, the fear of AIDS that exists in the general public is reflected in the attitudes of youth.

Attitudes of College Students

Findings for college students' fear of AIDS are contradictory but reconcilable. As noted previously, DiClemente et al. (1990) conducted an extensive survey of college students' knowledge and attitudes regarding AIDS and found that the level of students' knowledge about transmission routes was quite high. Yet 71% of the students reported that they were afraid of getting AIDS; 39% would feel afraid of getting AIDS from an infected student in class; 36% would feel afraid sitting in the same classroom as an infected student; and 41% would avoid getting too close to a gay male. Moreover, 25% of the respondents believed that students with AIDS should not be allowed to attend classes. These findings are essentially similar to those obtained for samples of high school students.

On the other hand, in separate studies, Simkins and his colleagues (Simkins & Eberhage, 1984; Simkins & Kushner, 1986) concluded that approximately 70% of the college students in their samples expressed no concern about AIDS. Two factors seem pertinent in attempting to reconcile these findings with those of DiClemente et al. (1990). First, the former studies were conducted several years earlier, and, as suggested by the results of Hingson et al. (1990), concern about AIDS has increased in recent years. Second, the fear of AIDS in the former studies was probably underestimated because the index was based on concern about contracting AIDS *from a present sexual partner*, rather than fear of AIDS in general.

Several investigators have examined the correlates of negative attitudes toward persons with AIDS in college students, and their findings are consistent with the contentions of Herek and Glunt (1988) noted previously. Triplet and Sugarman (1987) obtained respondents' ratings of personal responsibility and interactional desirability for eight hypothetical case descriptions that varied systematically on the client's sexual preference (homosexual or heterosexual) and diagnosis (AIDS, herpes, hepatitis, or Legionnaires' disease). Results showed that homosexuals were viewed as more personally responsible for their illness, irrespective of diagnosis. Persons with AIDS, especially homosexuals, received the lowest ratings on interactional desirability. The authors concluded that negative reactions against persons with AIDS reflect fear of the disease coupled with general prejudice against homosexuals. Consistent with this conclusion, Simkins and Kushner (1986) found that homophobia correlated positively with concern for AIDS, and Royse, Dhooper, and Hatch (1987) observed that empathy for persons with AIDS was associated inversely with fear of AIDS.

Attitudes of Health Care Professionals

Children with HIV receive their direct medical care from nurses, physicians, and other health care professionals. As such, the fears and concerns of these professionals may influence the quality of care and comfort provided to individuals with HIV. Although few investigators have assessed health care professionals' attitudes toward pediatric AIDS in particular, several studies have evaluated professionals' attitudes toward AIDS in general.

There is strong evidence that many health care professionals are extremely concerned about acquiring AIDS, view AIDS patients negatively, and feel emotional distress when working with AIDS patients. Imperato, Feldman, Nayeri, and DeHovitz (1988) found that a majority of second-year medical students perceived a definite risk of acquiring AIDS through patient contact, and, in spite of reaffirmations of legal and ethical responsibilities by professional organizations (e.g., American Medical Association, 1987), almost 50% of the students believed that physicians in private practice should have the prerogative of declining care for AIDS patients. Similarly, one half of the nurses in a study feared that AIDS could be contracted despite precautions (Blumenfield, Smith, Milazzo, Seropian, & Wormser, 1987), and almost half indicated that they would ask for a transfer if they had to care for AIDS patients on a regular basis. Such findings have been replicated with medical and pediatric interns and residents (Link, Feingold, Charap, Freeman, & Shelov, 1988). Finally, in a study that used standardized symptomatology inventories, Treiber, Shaw, and Malcolm (1987) concluded that nurses and physicians experienced increased anxiety, greater interference in nonwork activities, and more frequent negative rumination when working with AIDS patients than with non-AIDS patients.

Several well-designed studies have evaluated factors that contribute to fear of AIDS among health care professionals. Using vignettes that were identical in content except for the patient's sexual orientation and disease (AIDS vs. leukemia), Kelly, St. Lawrence, Smith, Hood, and Cook (1987a) assessed medical students' attitudes toward AIDS patients. Results showed that medical students viewed AIDS patients and homosexual patients very negatively, regardless of the latter's diagnosis. In another relatively sophisticated study, Pomerance and Shields (1989) used multiple regression analyses to determine the key predictors of hospital workers' perceived AIDS stress, AIDS comfort, and AIDS risk. Controlling for the effects of pertinent demographic characteristics and psychosocial variables, the researchers found that homophobia, transmission knowledge, and contact with AIDS patients contributed variance to each of the three dependent measures (i.e., AIDS stress, comfort, and risk). In addition, death anxiety contributed to AIDS-related stress. Similarly, O'Donnell, O'Donnell, Pleck, Snarey, and Rose (1987) reported high correlations among AIDS phobia, homophobia, and AIDS stress; and Royse and Birge (1987) demonstrated that homophobia was a significant predictor of fear of AIDS. Finally, in a sample of medical students and nursing students, Bliwise et al. (1991) found that negative attitudes toward AIDS were linked with homonegativism, prejudice against intravenous drug users, death anxiety, concerns about germs and disease, and beliefs about potential risk for AIDS. The investigators concluded that there are multiple pathways to negative attitudes toward AIDS patients.

Together, the results from these studies of health care professionals are congruent with Herek and Glunt's (1988) contention that negative attitudes toward AIDS reflect the danger of the disease as well as its association with stigmatized groups. As Gerbert and her colleagues have documented (Gerbert, Maguire, Badner, Altman, & Stone, 1989), health care professionals who come in contact with AIDS patients *are* at risk for exposure to HIV, and infection-control procedures do not always prevent needle sticks and other types of accidents. Moreover, it seems unrealistic to expect health care professionals to be any less prejudiced than other segments of society. Thus, as Gerbert and her colleagues conclude, such professionals should not be admonished for their fears. Finally, it remains to be determined whether health care professionals' fears of AIDS interfere with their actual caregiving behavior.

Summary and Conclusion

Several conclusions can be drawn from the literature regarding youths' knowledge, misconceptions, and attitudes about AIDS. First, extant research methodologies require considerable development and refinement. Second, the knowledge and attitudes of children have received scant attention. Third, in spite of methodological shortcomings, studies published recently indicate that adolescents and college students have high levels of knowledge about AIDS, though misconceptions regarding transmission routes persist. Fourth, adolescents and college students tend to hold negative attitudes toward AIDS and persons with AIDS, and such attitudes are probably associated with the deadly nature of the disease and the link between AIDS and groups of persons who are already stigmatized. The attitudes of adolescents and college students, however, are essentially similar to those held by the public and by health care professionals.

FOUR

Adolescent Sexual Behavior

Although few cases of AIDS have been reported for adolescents, it is estimated that young adults—most of whom were infected during adolescence—constitute approximately 20% of existing cases (Flora & Thoresen, 1989). The potential risk for adolescents is exacerbated by their high rates of risk-taking behaviors such as unprotected sexual intercourse and substance abuse. Likewise, adolescent females, who have a high pregnancy rate as a population, can transmit the virus to their offspring.

Hein (1989) has argued that there are important differences between adolescents and adults in sexual behavior and AIDS epidemiology that should be considered in planning appropriate responses to the AIDS epidemic. These differences are as follows:

1. A higher percentage of adolescent cases is acquired by heterosexual transmission.
2. A higher percentage of infected adolescents is asymptomatic.
3. A higher percentage of infected adolescents are minorities.
4. Special ethical and legal considerations pertain to minors (see Chapter 7).
5. Adolescents differ from adults in sociocognitive reasoning.
6. There are special economic and medical implications for infected adolescents who are pregnant.

7. Unified community support systems for infected adolescents are not available.

8. Adolescents as a population include a higher percentage of "sexual adventurers," who have many sexual contacts and rarely use contraceptives.

9. Convenient and appropriate health services are relatively unavailable for adolescents.

These differences between adolescents and adults, and their implications for the AIDS epidemic, will be discussed throughout this chapter. First, however, methodological concerns in researching the sexual behavior of adolescents will be briefly noted.

Methodological Considerations

Excellent overviews of problems in the study of sexual behavior have recently been published by Reinisch, Sanders, and Ziemba-Davis (1988) and Gagnon et al. (1989). The conclusions of these reviewers are summarized below regarding issues of construct validity, internal validity, and external validity.

Construct Validity

Gagnon et al. (1989) described several difficulties in the development of valid self-report instruments to measure sexual behavior. First, the accuracy of self-reports of sexual behavior rarely can be validated; for example, a surprisingly high percentage of participants in a longitudinal survey indicated that they were currently virgins, whereas the previous year they had reported experiencing sexual intercourse (Mott, 1985). Second, it is difficult to chose an appropriate time frame for rates of sexual behavior, and reliability of recall probably varies with the chosen time frame (e.g., previous 24 hours vs. previous 12 months). Third, behavioral specificity is an important prerequisite for measuring sexual behavior associated with HIV transmission. Such specificity, however, may be difficult to tap because of the naïveté of many adolescent respondents and the negative emotional response of the adolescents' parents to such specificity (i.e., the youth may be embarrassed, and the parents offended, by certain questions). Fourth, questionnaire items can be biased toward respondents of higher socioeconomic status (SES) and can be interpreted differently by different individuals.

In light of such problems with self-report instruments, Reinisch et al. (1988) concluded that interview methods provide more accurate data on sexual behavior. Interviewers can monitor respondents' reactions, tailor the vocabulary of questions, seek clarification of responses, normalize highly personal information, and respond immediately to distress. It is essential, however, that interview schedules be well standardized and that interviewers receive extensive training and possess requisite interpersonal skills. On the other hand, Gagnon et al. (1989) noted evidence that respondents are less likely to report sensitive sexual behavior during face-to-face contact than in anonymous surveys.

Internal Validity

Internal validity refers to the accuracy of associations that are observed between variables that represent underlying constructs. Assuming that construct validity is strong in a particular study, internal validity is limited most often by the researcher's failure to consider alternative explanations (i.e., third variables) for observed associations between variables and/or possible mediators of such associations. The investigation of third variables and mediators of associations characterize more highly developed areas of research on adolescent behavior (e.g., multivariate causal models of antisocial behavior in adolescents; Henggeler, 1991). In contrast, studies of adolescent sexual behavior tend to be descriptive or to evaluate simple zero-order correlations between variables.

External Validity

The vast majority of research on adolescent sexual behavior has used convenience samples (Gagnon et al, 1989; Reinisch et al., 1988). Exceptions include the large national surveys described by Zelnik and his colleagues. The focus of these surveys, however, was on issues associated with adolescent pregnancy, rather than on the delineation of adolescent sexual behavior per se. Thus the surveys included relatively little information regarding rates and types of specific sexual practices among adolescents.

TABLE 4.1   Percentage of 15- to 19-Year-Old Adolescent Women Who Had Premarital Sexual Intercourse

	1971	1976	1979	1982
White	26	38	47	43
African-American	54	66	66	54
Total	30	43	50	45

Sexual Behavior of Adolescents

Adolescent sexual behavior must be conceptualized within its broader systemic context. That is, such behavior covaries with other types of "acting-out" behaviors, such as substance use and delinquency (e.g., Jessor & Jessor, 1977). Moreover, adolescent sexual behavior, substance use, and delinquency share common correlates. Each is linked with similar adolescent cognitive characteristics, family relations, peer associations, and school performance, as noted in this chapter and in Chapter 5. As discussed in Chapter 6, the covariation of these problems may require preventive strategies that are comprehensive and that possess the flexibility for selective intensity (Melton, 1988a).

Heterosexual Behavior

The most extensive data regarding adolescent sexual activity have been obtained in a series of national household (and sometimes dormitory) surveys (Hofferth, Kahn, & Baldwin, 1987; Zelnik & Kantner, 1980; Zelnik & Shah, 1983). As shown in Table 4.1, there are two interesting longitudinal trends in the percentages of urban 15- to 19-year-old adolescent women who have had premarital sexual intercourse. First, the percentage is higher among African-American adolescents than among white adolescents. Second, the percentages have stabilized and even may have declined, especially for African-American women. Nevertheless, Hofferth et al. (1987) concluded that, across racial groups, adolescents are becoming sexually experienced at younger and younger ages.

Zelnik and Shah (1983), based on a 1979 survey, found race and gender differences in the age of adolescents' first intercourse as well as gender and age differences in the nature of the youths' first sexual partner. African-American females were approximately 1 year younger than their white counterparts (15.5 years vs. 16.4 years) when they first experienced intercourse; similarly, African-American males were 1.5 years younger than their white counterparts (14.4 years vs. 15.9 years). Regarding characteristics of the adolescents' first sexual partner, males tended to have their first intercourse with females of similar age, whereas females tended to have their first intercourse with males who were 3 years older, on the average. Moreover, females were more likely than males to feel an emotional commitment to their first partner, and youths who had their first sexual intercourse at an older age were more likely to feel an emotional commitment to their partner than were their younger counterparts.

If it is assumed that earlier initiation of sexual activity and less familiarity with one's sexual partners are risk factors for HIV transmission, then the preceding data suggest that urban African-American male adolescents are at relatively high risk (irrespective of condom use, which will be discussed shortly). The high-risk status of this population is supported further by the results of a survey of inner-city African-American male adolescents attending junior high school or senior high school in Baltimore (Clark, Zabin, & Hardy, 1984). Sixty-five percent of the adolescents reported to have had their first sexual experience before the age of 13 years, and the senior high school males reported an average of six sexual contacts during the preceding month.

African-American male adolescents are certainly not the only group of youths who are at increased risk of HIV infection because of their high rates of sexual activity. Sorensen (1973), in a national survey of adolescents, concluded that 41% of sexually active males and 13% of sexually active females were characterized as "sexual adventurers" (i.e., they had numerous sexual partners over relatively brief periods of time).

Correlates of heterosexual activity. The correlates of early sexual activity in adolescents parallel those of adolescent criminal behavior (Henggeler, 1989) and adolescent substance use (see Chapter 5). Moreover, these correlates are consistent with social-ecological models of behavior (e.g., Bronfenbrenner, 1979). In other words, adolescent sexual behavior is associated with multiple characteristics of the individual youth and of the social systems in which he or she is embedded (Voydanoff & Donnelly, 1990). There are complex interrelations among these characteristics, and the contextual variables often contribute more variance than do biological and individual variables.

As reviewed by Brooks-Gunn and Furstenberg (1989) and Voydanoff and Donnelly (1990), *biological* variables such as hormonal activation and physical maturity interact with social context to influence sexual behavior. In addition, the average age of biological maturity has declined during recent decades, and such decline increases the propensity for sexual activity at a time when the youth's cognitive and emotional development is relatively immature. *Individual* characteristics such as attitudes toward sexuality, attitudes toward nonmarital intercourse, and social cognitive reasoning are linked with sexual activity. Pertinent *family* correlates of sexual activity include demographic characteristics such as socioeconomic status, family size, and family structure, as well as qualitative variables such as parent-adolescent communication, family affect and support, and parental supervision.

Extrafamilial correlates of sexual activity pertain primarily to peer, school, and societal influences. Sexual activity is linked with *peer* pressure and perceived peer sexual activity. Regarding *school*, sexual activity is associated with low intellectual ability, low educational goals, and poor school performance. At the *societal level*, technological advancements (e.g., telephones, cars, contraception) have provided more opportunities for sexual activity by increasing the autonomy of adolescents. Moreover, these technological changes have coincided with a societal shift in the direction of a less restrictive attitude toward nonmarital sexual activity. Together, these findings support a multicausal view of adolescent sexual activity. This view is supported further by investigations that have used multivariate analyses (e.g., Gibbs, 1986).

Homosexuality

Gagnon et al. (1989) noted several dimensions of sexual behavior between persons of the same gender that are relevant to the sexual transmission of HIV: (a) the percentage of the population that engages in such sexual relations, (b) the frequency of such contacts and the number of different partners, (c) the sexual techniques that are used, (d) the number of sexual partners of the opposite gender, and (e) the social characteristics and other sexual relations of the sexual partners. Gagnon and his colleagues provide an excellent review of these dimensions as they pertain to adult homosexuality. There are scant data, unfortunately, regarding the sexual behavior of adolescents who have sexual relations with persons of the same gender (Brooks-Gunn & Furstenberg, 1989).

Recent research findings suggest, however, that gay adolescents are at unusually high risk for HIV transmission. Remafedi (1987a) assessed 29 self-identified homosexual or bisexual adolescent males who were recruited through advertisements. The sample was predominantly white and middle-class. High percentages of the youths had serious emotional and behavioral problems, including substance abuse (58%), conflict with the law (48%), sexually transmitted diseases (45%), suicide attempts (34%), dropping out of high school (28%), and prostitution (17%). Moreover, when questioned about their most recent homosexual contacts, the youths reported that they knew their partner for more than a week in only 28% of cases. Meetings in gay bars and public places accounted for the majority of encounters. Although the external validity of these findings may be low, the results certainly suggest that gay youths are in jeopardy for HIV transmission because of both the nature of their sexual relations and the high prevalence of other types of problems that are risk factors (Remafedi, 1988).

Sexually Transmitted Diseases (STDs)

Prevalence data for STDs are further indication that adolescents are at relatively high risk for AIDS. When prevalence data are based on the proportion of sexually active individuals, 10- to 14-year-olds and 15- to 19-year-olds have the highest rates of gonorrhea, syphilis, and chlamydia in the population (Bell & Hein, 1984). Likewise, a relatively high percentage of adolescents harbor asymptomatic STDs (Hein, 1987a). Risk factors for STDs include an early age of intercourse and minimal contraceptive use (Brooks-Gunn, Boyer, & Hein, 1988).

Contraceptive Use

Based on findings from surveys conducted by Zelnik and his colleagues, Brooks-Gunn and Furstenberg (1989) noted in their review of adolescent sexual behavior that the high incidence of adolescent pregnancy in the United States, relative to other industrialized nations, is partly the product of poor contraceptive use among American youths. For example, Zelnik and Shah (1983) examined reports of the contraceptive method used at first intercourse by females aged 15 to 19 years and males aged 17 to 21 years. Even when the first intercourse was planned, only 72% of the females reported using contraception, and only 51% of the males reported such use. Moreover, when the first intercourse was not planned, these figures decrease to 44% and 42%, respectively. Although condoms were usually the most commonly used method for both males and females, condoms were used only about 20% of the time in instances of first intercourse (planned or unplanned). African-American youths were less likely than their white counterparts to use contraception in general, and condoms in particular. When asked why they did not use contraception, male and female respondents who had planned their first intercourse indicated that they (a) did not want to use contraceptives, (b) did not know about contraception, (c) did not think about using contraceptives, (d) thought that pregnancy was impossible, and/or (e) did not have access to contraception. In addition to these reasons, approximately 25% of the youths who did not plan their first intercourse indicated that their failure to use contraception was attributable to the spontaneity of the circumstance.

The preceding results, based on data collected before the AIDS epidemic, suggest that during their first intercourse youths rarely use a contraceptive method that is an effective barrier to HIV infection. Perhaps, however, such contraception is used more frequently in subsequent sexual activity. Zelnik and Kantner (1980) surveyed contraceptive use among sexually active 15- to 19-year-old females and found that more than 25% reported that they never used contraception. Of those that did use contraception, only 23% used condoms. On the positive side, however, adolescent females who had received sex education were more likely to use contraception than their counterparts who had not had sex education (Zelnik & Kim, 1982). If current adolescent contraception use is similar to practices reported in the 1970s, the spread of HIV through the adolescent population should be a significant concern. Recent surveys of adolescent sexual activity and condom use will be reviewed shortly.

Correlates of contraceptive use. The correlates of irregular contraceptive use in adolescent females are similar to the correlates of sexual activity, substance use, and other antisocial behavior. Reviewers

(Brooks-Gunn & Furstenberg, 1989; Morrison, 1985; Voydanoff & Donnelly, 1990) have concluded that poor contraceptive use in female adolescents is associated with multiple characteristics of the adolescents and of the social systems in which they are embedded.

Several individual characteristics of the women are linked with irregular contraceptive use, including young age (and less cognitive maturity), inadequate knowledge about reproduction and contraception, low self-esteem, high anxiety, and feelings of alienation. Family relationship variables associated with irregular contraceptive use include low parental support, poor family communication, and parent-adolescent conflict. In the area of sexual partner correlates, women with greater interpersonal influence and couples with more open communication are more likely to use contraceptives reliably. Friendships with problem peers and difficulties in school also have been linked with irregular contraceptive use. Little is known about the contraceptive use of male adolescents.

Effects of Sex Education
and Other Prevention Programs

In reviewing the effects of sex education, it should be remembered that *sex education* is a generic term for a diverse range of educational interventions and that the implementation of such programs is far from universal (Brooks-Gunn & Furstenberg, 1989). For example, in a survey of sex-education teachers, Forrest and Silverman (1989) found that only 52% provided information about sources of birth control and only 70% covered homosexuality. Similarly, sex education in Canada is provided in 87% of urban school districts, but only 25% of rural school districts (Herold, Fisher, Smith, & Yarber, 1990).

Given the considerable national debate regarding the merits of sex education, there are surprisingly few evaluations of its effects on adolescents' sexual activity. Based on a national household survey of 15- and 16-year-olds, Furstenberg, Moore, and Peterson (1985) concluded that sex education was associated with a 33% reduction in the prevalence of sexual intercourse. The size of this reduction was maintained when the effects of socioeconomic status were statistically controlled, and the reductions held for race (African-American vs. white) and gender groups, with the exception of

African-American males. Because African-American males tend to initiate sexual intercourse at a relatively young age, the authors posited that sex education may have been offered too late to influence their behavior. On the other hand, Zelnik and Kim (1982) concluded that sex education was not associated with the prevalence of sexual intercourse among female adolescents participating in their national survey. Sex education, however, was linked with lower rates of pregnancy and with a higher probability of contraception use at first intercourse. Similarly, Brooks-Gunn and Furstenberg (1989) noted that some school-based family-planning clinics have produced a delay of first intercourse, increased use of contraception, and decreased pregnancy rates.

Voydanoff and Donnelly (1990) reviewed other types of interventions aimed at decreasing sexual activity and increasing contraceptive use. Family communication programs have shown increases in family discussions about sexuality, but long-term effects have not been demonstrated. Similarly, peer counseling programs and media-oriented programs have little empirical support for their efficacy. In light of the multicausal nature of sexual activity and contraceptive use, broad-based and comprehensive interventions approaches might be expected to enhance prevention efficacy. Indeed, Voydanoff and Donnelly concluded that such multifaceted programs (e.g., integrating educational, vocational, counseling, and health care services) hold the most promise.

Sexual Behavior
Since the AIDS Epidemic

Investigators have begun to study the effect of the AIDS epidemic on the sexual behavior of adolescents and college students. Although the researchers almost always indicated that their study examined the "impact" of AIDS on sexual behavior or "changes" in sexual behavior, it must be noted that, with one exception, each of these studies is cross-sectional and that the evaluation of behavior change requires a longitudinal design. Nevertheless, the following findings are quite heuristic and provide a disconcerting comparison with the survey data collected during the 1970s.

62   PEDIATRIC AND ADOLESCENT AIDS

High School Students

   Kegeles et al. (1988) used a longitudinal design and surveyed 204
adolescents who attended an HMO in San Francisco. The investigators found no evidence that rates of condom use had increased during
the 14 months between the two surveys. Although sexually active
adolescents valued condoms highly as a protection against STDs,
only 2% of females and 8% of males reported using condoms during
every intercourse in the previous year. Moreover, the females reported minimal intention ever to use condoms.
   Hingson and his colleagues (Hingson, Strunin, & Berlin, 1990;
Hingson, Strunin, Berlin, & Heeren, 1990) conducted independent
statewide phone surveys of adolescents living in Massachusetts in
1986 and 1988. Results from the 1988 survey suggested that a greater
percentage (19% vs. 2%) of adolescents reported adopting condom
use because of AIDS than in 1986. A high degree of response bias,
however, was probably evoked by the nature of certain questions
(e.g., "Have you adopted condom use because of AIDS?"), and such
bias should be expected to interact with the respondents' degree of
knowledge about the disease (which also increased in 1988). In the
1988 survey, 31% of sexually active youths indicated that they
always used condoms, 32% reported that they sometimes used condoms, and 37% indicated that they never used condoms. Condoms
were least likely to be used by adolescents who reported only one
sexual partner during the previous year, and substance use was associated with a lower probability of condom use. Moreover, 18% of all
respondents indicated that they had unprotected intercourse with
more than one partner in the previous years. Unfortunately, the
authors did not report comparable data from the 1986 survey.
   Several surveys of relatively high-risk female adolescents have
been conducted in family-planning clinics. Weisman et al. (1989) used
multiple regression analysis to assess the variables most closely
associated with condom use at last intercourse. The only significant
predictor of condom use was having had previous experience in
asking a partner to use a condom. Condom use was not associated
with perceived risk of AIDS or with knowing that condom use reduces
the AIDS risk. Seltzer et al. (1989), using an assessment strategy with
a high degree of response bias, asked whether and how female
adolescent respondents had changed their sexual practices since
hearing about AIDS. Fifty-nine percent of the youths indicated that

they had changed their sexual behavior (e.g., fewer partners, less frequent intercourse, more frequent use of condoms). Finally, Beaman and Strader (1989) evaluated a sample of STD patients that included a high percentage of adolescents. Participants were knowledgeable about AIDS and about the role of condoms in reducing the risk of HIV infection. Yet only 30% of the respondents were presently using condoms, and in that group, condoms were used in only 25% of sexual encounters.

Together, the results from recent studies of adolescent sexual behavior and condom use do little to ease the concern raised by surveys conducted in the 1970s. It is admittedly difficult to contrast the findings of studies that use widely different methods and assess diverse samples. Nevertheless, it seems quite clear that a great many adolescents engage in unsafe sexual activity, and that they engage in this activity in spite of having high levels of knowledge about AIDS and about the value of condoms in protecting against HIV infection.

College Students

In light of the greater cognitive maturity of college students (at least relative to high school students) and the association between social cognition and sexual behavior/contraception use, one would expect that college students engage in relatively low rates of unsafe sexual activity. The extant data, however, do not support this expectation. Strader and Beaman (1989) surveyed a convenience sample of midwestern college students and found that 60% of the students were presently sexually active, and that 21% had been active previously. Yet, in spite of the fact that 96% of the sample knew that condom use lowers the risk of HIV transmission, only 40% of the sexually experienced young adults had ever used a condom. The reluctance of college students to use condoms was probably linked with negative beliefs about condom use (e.g., that condom use decreases pleasure for self and partner, that it is inconvenient and uncomfortable).

Similar findings of risky behavior among college students were reported by Baldwin and Baldwin (1988). Among sexually active respondents, the average number of sexual partners during the past 3 months was 1.5, and 19% of the young adults had engaged in sexual intercourse with a stranger or a casual acquaintance. In spite of high levels of knowledge about AIDS, condom use was relatively infrequent, with only 13% of the students always using condoms and 66% never using condoms. Correlates of condom use included high socioeconomic status, Hispanic ethnicity, older age of first intercourse, and regular use of seat belts (probably indicating less willingness to take risks). Condom use was not associated with cognitive variables such as knowledge about HIV transmission, perceived AIDS risk, or worry about contracting AIDS.

The findings from these convenience samples are consistent with the findings from a large multisite, cross-sectional survey of college students (DiClemente et al., 1990). Eighty-two percent of the sample was sexually active, with 16% reporting 11 or more sexual contacts and 4% reporting receptive anal intercourse during the previous month. In addition, students were very knowledgeable about AIDS and the role of condoms in preventing HIV transmission. Nevertheless, 37% of the respondents never used condoms during intercourse, and only 8% reported that they always used condoms. Knowledge about AIDS was not associated with reported changes in condom use, though perceived risk for contracting AIDS was linked with such reported changes. Finally, Fisher and Misovich (1990) surveyed convenience samples of college students in three successive years and concluded that certain risky sexual practices had become more common in spite of increased knowledge about AIDS and more favorable attitudes toward safe sex. In summary, findings regarding condom use among college students are similar to those described for younger adolescents. Despite high levels of knowledge about AIDS and safe sex practices, condom use is infrequent.

Barriers to Changing Sexual Behavior

Melton (1988a) and Siegel and Gibson (1988) have delineated several obstacles to decreasing risky sexual behavior in adolescents and young adults. First, the widespread emphases on homosexual anal intercourse and intravenous drug use as primary modes of HIV transmission may have led heterosexual youths to feel largely invulnerable to AIDS. Second, although knowledge about AIDS does not seems to be linked to sexual activities in adolescents, it is important that youths have accurate knowledge about sex, contraception, and AIDS. Such knowledge is certainly necessary, though not sufficient, for effective behavior change. Third, youths' beliefs and attitudes about condoms militate against their use. For example, condoms are often viewed as uncomfortable, an impediment to erotic love-making, embarrassing to purchase, and an indication of promiscuity.

Fourth, adolescent sexual behavior is associated with perceived peer group norms, and such norms often account for more variance in the behavior of adolescents than do cognitive variables. Thus successful interventions may need to target complex social systems as well as youths' knowledge, attitudes, and beliefs. Fifth, in light of the interpersonal nature of sexual intercourse, it is also necessary to have the communication and assertion skills needed to "negotiate" safe sex with a partner. The development of effective communication skills regarding emotionally sensitive and/or embarrassing issues such as condom use and STDs will not be easy for many adolescents to achieve. Sixth, the stigma of AIDS and other STDs makes it difficult to seek out information from a sexual partner. In the passion of the moment, few adolescents are willing to risk rejection by asking their partner about his or her risk history. Suggestions for overcoming these obstacles are outlined in Chapter 6.

Cultural factors. Several reviewers have addressed cultural factors that may be pertinent to the reduction of risky sexual behavior in minorities (e.g., Mays & Cochran, 1988; Peterson & Marin, 1988; Schilling et al., 1989; Schinke, Botvin, Orlandi, Schilling, & Gordon, 1990). As noted earlier, there are cultural differences in factors such as age of first intercourse and prevalence of contraception use. To the best of our knowledge, however, few data suggest that the correlates and causes of risky sexual behavior are different for whites than for African-Americans and Hispanic-Americans. If this is the case, interventions targeted at minorities may need to be more intensive than those targeted at whites, but the qualitative nature of the interventions may be quite similar (aside from superficial differences in language used and social context displayed). On the other hand, there is some evidence of cultural differences in sexual relations that would require special consideration of culture. For example, Peterson and Marin (1988) noted that there are few formal gay organizations in minority communities, and, consequently, interventions that have relied on such organizations to reach white gay men will not be effective for reaching their minority counterparts. Cultural factors are discussed more extensively in Chapter 5.

Summary

A brief review of the correlates of adolescent sexual activity and contraceptive use indicated that these variables are linked with characteristics of the adolescents and of the social systems in which they are embedded (family, peer, school), and that these correlates are quite similar to those identified for adolescent antisocial behavior and substance use (see Chapter 5). Such findings suggest that broad-based preventive efforts may be more viable than efforts that focus on only one aspect of the youths' ecology. Surveys of sexual activity among high school students and among college students conducted since the AIDS epidemic indicate that a high percentage of youths engages in unsafe sexual activity in spite of having a high level of knowledge about AIDS and about the value of condoms in protecting against HIV infection. Barriers to changing sexual behavior were noted; suggestions for overcoming these barriers are outlined in Chapter 6.

FIVE

Adolescent Intravenous Drug Use

Intravenous (IV) drug use is associated with transmission of HIV in three ways (Leukefeld, Battjes, & Amsel, 1990). First, and most frequent for IV drug users, HIV is spread through the sharing of contaminated drug injection equipment. Such sharing led to an HIV infection rate of over 60% among IV drug abusers in New York City. Second, the virus can be transmitted during sexual relations between IV drug users and their partners. This mode of transmission has accounted for approximately 70% of cases of AIDS in the United States attributed to heterosexual activity. Third, HIV can be transmitted perinatally by women who are IV drug users or whose partners are IV drug users. Perinatal transmission has accounted for 75% of AIDS cases in young children.

After methodological considerations are discussed, several areas of research regarding the transmission of the disease by IV drug users will be reviewed. These areas include ethnographic studies of the social context of IV drug use, multivariate studies of adolescent substance abuse, studies of the sexual behavior of IV drug users, issues of particular significance to IV drug-abusing women and minorities, and research on behavioral changes among IV drug users since the AIDS epidemic.

Methodological Considerations

In an overview of the link between IV drug use and AIDS, Barker et al. (1989) noted several significant methodological concerns. Regarding external validity, extant knowledge about IV drug use has been derived primarily from convenience samples of adults obtained from correctional facilities and treatment centers. Findings based on these samples may not generalize to subgroups of adolescent IV drug users. For example, Mata and Jorquez (1989) reported that young Mexican-American IV drug users had very different patterns of use than did their older counterparts. Younger IV drug users were less aware of health risk factors and were less cautious about sharing their drugs and drug injection equipment.

The primary reason that investigators have focused on "captive" samples is the extreme difficulty in conducting surveys with deviant subcultures. Such subcultures are usually closed to outsiders, and the members quite justifiably fear exposure of their illegal activities. Consequently, ethnographic field researchers have provided most of our existing knowledge about the behaviors of IV drug-using subcultures (e.g., Oetting, Edwards, & Beauvais, 1989). Data from qualitative studies often provide rich sources of information from which hypotheses can be generated.

Another impediment to conducting research with IV drug users is the construct validity of the self-report instruments. Although results from ethnographic studies can be used to improve the wording of survey instruments, many respondents may not have the requisite literacy or facility in spoken English. Similarly, related issues of internal validity pertain to the deliberate falsification of responses. Respondents often are hesitant to provide accurate information about their illegal activities, or they might exaggerate these activities. Further complicating the acquisition of valid data is the distortion of memory and inaccurate recall of past events associated with substance abuse. In spite of these many problems, the validity of findings from self-report surveys is supported in both the general substance abuse literature (e.g., Dembo et al., 1987) and by observed associations between the reported frequency of sharing drug injection equipment and the risk of HIV infection (Robertson, Bucknall, & Welsby, 1986).

Mechanics and Frequency of IV Drug Use

As Barker et al. (1989) noted, *needle sharing* is a shorthand term that encompasses several ways in which HIV can be transmitted through the sharing of drug injection equipment. Contamination with infected blood that remains in the syringe probably accounts for the heaviest doses of HIV. HIV transmission can also occur, however, when (a) infected blood remains inside or outside the needle, (b) the process of drawing up the drug solution contaminates the small container (e.g., a spoon) on which the drug was dissolved, (c) cotton used to strain out impurities from the drug solution becomes contaminated, or (d) contaminated injection equipment is washed with water that serves as a common rinse source.

The probability of becoming seropositive varies with the frequency of injection with contaminated equipment and consequent exposure to varying doses of HIV (Barker et al., 1989). There are wide individual variations in patterns of IV drug use. Some IV drug users are hard-core addicts who inject several times per day, whereas others are occasional recreational drug users. In addition, many IV drug users inject multiple drugs, and different drugs are associated with different frequencies of injection. For example, cocaine is injected more frequently than heroin because of its relatively short-lived effects. It also seems that the choice of drugs and drug injection practices can vary considerably among different drug subcultures and at different points in time. Thus, for any particular IV drug user, there are several variables that influence the HIV dosage to which he or she may been exposed.

Prevalence and Social Context of IV Drug Use

Based on national estimates that have considerable error variance (Barker et al., 1989), there are approximately 900,000 regular users of IV drugs (i.e., persons injecting at least once per week) and 200,000 occasional users. The overall seroprevalence rates for regular users and occasional users are estimated at 25% and 5%, respectively, although there is much regional variation in these rates. For example, 55% of drug-related AIDS cases occurred in the Northeast (CDC, 1989).

The prevalence of IV drug use among adolescents is difficult to discern. In their 1988 statewide survey of 1,762 adolescents in Massachusetts, Hingson, Strunin, and Berlin (1990) found that only 0.1% of the youths reported IV drug use. Similarly, in the National Youth Survey, fewer than 1% of youths reported heroin use during the past year (Elliott, Ageton, Huizinga, Knowles, & Canter, 1983). National surveys such as these, however, probably underestimate the prevalence of IV drug use in adolescents because high-risk subgroups (e.g., incarcerated juvenile offenders, homeless youths) are not included in the samples.

Qualitative interviews indicate that the IV drug user's first injection experience often is recalled fondly (Ingold & Ingold, 1989). The first injection usually is performed by friends with whom the user has a history of drug taking. These friends teach the proper techniques for handling the syringe and needle, and they provide the user with emotional and social support for the negative side effects of the injection (e.g., nausea). The social context of the initiation to IV drug use contributes to the notion that such drug use is a communal activity (Barker et al., 1989).

In addition to the social context of the first injection experience, there are several other reasons why sharing drug injection equipment has been common in the IV drug-using subculture. Sharing may reflect the social bonding among "running partners" who cooperate to obtain drugs and the money needed to purchase them (Des Jarlais & Friedman, 1987a). Sharing drug injection equipment also has economic advantages; because of legal restrictions, it may be difficult and costly to obtain a stable supply of sterile needles and syringes (Peterson & Marin, 1988). Moreover, to some extent, the group can protect drug users from the violence of the subculture and from exposure to law enforcement officers (Barker et al., 1989). Pertinent to the IV drug use of adolescents, investigators have reported that the sharing of drug injection equipment is most frequent among younger users (Ginzburg et al., 1986).

Social-Ecological Context of Adolescent Substance Abuse

Although there is scant research examining the causes and correlates of IV drug use in adolescents, there is an emerging literature examining the causes and correlates of adolescent substance abuse.

One of the consistent findings in this literature is that the causes and correlates of adolescent substance abuse are highly similar to those identified for antisocial youth behavior in general. Overwhelming empirical evidence (for comprehensive reviews, see Henggeler, 1989; Kazdin, 1987; Melton & Hargrove, in press; Quay, 1987) indicates that general antisocial behavior is related to important characteristics of the individual youth (e.g., moral reasoning, self-esteem), family (e.g., warmth, parental discipline skills, parental deviance), peer system (e.g, association with deviant peers), and school system (e.g., academic performance). Likewise, adolescent substance abuse has been associated with youth characteristics such as assertion/social skills (Botvin, Baker, Botvin, Filazzola, & Millman, 1984; Wills, Baker, & Botvin, 1989), expectancies (Christiansen, Smith, Roehling, & Goldman, 1989), and depression (Joshi & Scott, 1988); family factors such as family affective relations and parental support (Barrett, Simpson, & Lehman, 1988; Huba, Wingard, & Bentler, 1980) and parental deviance (Brook, Whiteman, & Gordon, 1983; Halebsky, 1987); peer factors such as association with deviant peers and conformity to peer pressure (Kandel, 1980; Oetting & Beauvais, 1990); and school factors such as poor academic performance and dropping out (Mills & Noyes, 1984).

Given the numerous correlates of general antisocial behavior, several research groups (e.g., Agnew, 1985; Elliott, Huizinga, & Ageton, 1985) have developed empirically based multidimensional causal models (for a review, see Henggeler, 1991). Across studies, there was consistent support for the view that variance is contributed directly or indirectly by variables at the youth, family, peer, and school levels. Likewise, several groups of investigators have developed multidimensional models of adolescent substance use. For example, Elliott et al. (1985) found that substance use was predicted directly from previous substance use and association with deviant peers; levels of family bonding and school bonding predicted association with deviant peers. Swaim, Oetting, Edwards, and Beauvais (1989) found that drug use was predicted directly by association with drug-using peers and that emotional distress had a small effect on associating with drug-using peers (family and school variables were not examined). Rhodes and Jason (1990) concluded that the level of family functioning was the most powerful predictor of substance abuse and that the youth's assertion skills also contributed unique variance. Finally, using an approach that is similar to causal modeling,

Johnson et al. (1990) found that personal, peer, and family factors contributed to substance use. Together, the findings from these studies and from those that model delinquency explicate the multidimensional nature of antisocial behavior.

The view that substance abuse can be linked with characteristics of individual youths and of the social systems in which they are embedded is consistent with the suppositions of systemic/social-ecological theories of child development and behavior (e.g., Bronfenbrenner, 1979; Henggeler & Borduin, 1990). Moreover, as discussed later in this volume, the multidimensional nature of substance abuse has important implications for the design of intervention and prevention strategies.

Drug Use, Sexual Behavior, and Women's Issues

There is a positive association between adolescent substance use and sexual activity (Jessor & Jessor, 1977). This association reflects the interrelations that often are observed among different types of antisocial behavior in adolescents. It seems, however, that adolescent substance use also is associated with a decreased probability of using condoms during sexual intercourse. Hingson and his colleagues (Hingson, Strunin, Berlin, & Heeren, 1990) found relatively low rates of condom use among adolescents who drank heavily or smoked marijuana. Moreover, compared with other sexually active adolescents who used substances, those who used condoms less often after substance use tended to be younger, to have less knowledge and more misconceptions about AIDS, and to have more sexual partners. Thus those adolescent substance users at the greatest risk of HIV infection took the fewest precautions.

Barker et al. (1989) drew several conclusions that pertain to HIV transmission in their review of the sexual activity of IV drug users. First, the majority of male IV drug users are in primary relationships with women who do not use drugs. On the other hand, female IV drug users are almost always paired with male IV drug users (Des Jarlais, Chamberland, Yancovitz, Weinberg, & Friedman, 1984). These latter women are at risk of infection both from their partners and from sharing drug injection equipment. Second, it is extremely difficult for IV drug-using women to request changes in sexual practices, because these women fear that such requests would jeopardize their personal, financial, and drug needs (Wofsy, 1987). Third, there is an association between drug use and promiscuity and prostitution (E. M. Johnson, 1987), and female IV drug users may be poor users of contraception (Ralph & Spigner, 1986).

The special problems faced by women IV drug users have been addressed by several investigators (e.g., Karan, 1989; Mondanaro, 1987). As Karan (1989) noted, slightly more than one half of women with AIDS are IV drug users (CDC, 1989), and 90% of these women are of childbearing age. Although rates of HIV infection attributable to homosexual activity are decreasing, there are increasing numbers of HIV infections in IV drug-using women and their newborns (see Chapter 2). In addition, several cofactors increase the risk for AIDS in women who are IV drug users (Mondanaro, 1987), including poor nutrition, drug-induced suppression of the immune system, repeated bouts of infection, high stress, and low prevention motivation.

Karan (1989) argued that several factors contribute to the spread of HIV in such women and their newborns. First, increased sexual freedom has led to earlier sexual activity and more numerous sexual partners. Second, birth control is usually viewed as the woman's responsibility, and most IV drug-using women have great difficulty negotiating sexual practices. Third, there has been a shift away from using condoms, because of complaints by male partners. Women IV drug users are often passive and fear that demands on partners to follow safer sex practices may lead to abandonment and economic loss. Moreover, for many women, sexuality is one of the main ways to experience and to maintain intimacy (Karan, 1989; Mondanaro, 1987). Fourth, motherhood is an important value in many cultures, and abortion often is prohibited. Fifth, IV drug-using women are more likely to prostitute themselves to procure drugs.

The life situations of IV drug-using women infected with HIV who become pregnant are especially difficult (Karan, 1989). Aside from the many psychosocial and economic difficulties associated with their drug use, these women experience grief attributable to their loss of health and the jeopardy of their infants (Wofsy, 1987). Their serious social and economic problems are exacerbated by their lack of social support networks, social isolation, and by AIDS-related stigma. Additionally, because of poor health and frequent abdication of child-rearing responsibility by the father, IV drug-using mothers often are unable to care for their children, and the children subsequently are placed in hospitals and foster homes.

Cultural Effects

African-Americans and Hispanic-Americans are represented disproportionately in the populations of both IV drug users and AIDS cases. These minorities account for about 40% of all AIDS cases, and nearly half of these cases have occurred among heterosexual IV drug users and their sexual partners (Peterson & Marin, 1988). Moreover, African-Americans account for approximately 80% of heterosexual transmission cases in men and 53% in women (Mays, 1989). The high prevalence of HIV among minority IV drug users is responsible for the disproportionate percentage of seropositive children who are minorities (75%).

Although the high prevalence of AIDS among Hispanic-Americans and African-Americans is attributable in part to the relatively high prevalence of IV drug use in these populations, minority IV drug users are more likely to be seropositive than are their white counterparts (Schilling et al., 1989). As Schilling and his colleagues observed, however, there are no ready biological or behavioral explanations for these cultural differences in seroprevalence. Some investigators have found higher rates of drug equipment sharing among minorities than among whites, but other researchers have reported opposite findings or no between-groups effects.

Although the prevalence of IV drug use is higher among African-Americans and Hispanic-Americans than among whites, little evidence suggests that the causes and correlates of substance abuse are different for these minorities than for whites. Analogously, the correlates of antisocial behavior are the same for boys as for girls, despite considerable gender differences in rates of antisocial behavior (Henggeler, 1989). Boys are simply more likely to evidence deficits on the variables linked with antisocial behavior. Likewise, the paths to IV drug use are probably the same for minorities as for whites, but minorities are more likely to experience difficulties on risk factors such as family relations and success in school. This position is consistent with the contention that the influences of substance abuse itself and the social context of such abuse outweigh possible cultural differences among abusers (Schilling et al., 1989). Nevertheless, theorists have argued uniformly for the importance of ethnic sensitivity in the design of interventions.

Mays (1989) identified several aspects of African-American culture that should be considered in the design of preventive interventions.

First, the church is the moral and social foundation of many African-American communities, and interventions should fit the values of the often fundamentalist religion. Second, relative to whites, African-Americans watch more television, give greater credibility to television as a source of information, and are more likely to rely on television as a primary source of news. Mays points out that major corporations have been very successful at using television and other avenues (e.g., billboards, sponsoring community events) to influence the buying habits of African-Americans. Third, African-Americans tend to maintain frequent contact with both immediate and extended family, and this kin network provides much tangible and social support (Mays & Cochran, 1987). Fourth, many African-Americans belong to a difficult-to-reach underclass of citizens who are frustrated, angry, and have many psychosocial difficulties. These individuals, who are probably at greatest risk of infection, will be the hardest to influence. In light of these cultural variables, Orlandi (1986) has argued that interventions should be primarily family-based and delivered in community settings (e.g., church) rather than in institutional settings such as schools. Our treatment research in the area of antisocial behavior (Brunk, Henggeler, & Whelan, 1987; Henggeler, Melton, & Smith, in press; Henggeler et al., 1986) strongly supports the viability of home-based and family-based interventions in multiproblem, minority families.

There is considerable cultural diversity among the different groups of Hispanic-Americans (Ruiz, 1985). For example, Cuban-Americans emigrated to the United States primarily from urban areas and for political reasons. In contrast, Puerto Ricans and Mexican-Americans emigrated primarily for economic reasons, and many of these first-generation Americans return periodically to their homelands. There are also differences in substance use: Heroin addiction is relatively prevalent among Puerto Ricans, cocaine abuse is relatively prevalent among Cuban-Americans, and inhalant use is relatively prevalent among Mexican-American adolescents (Orlandi, 1986).

There are several aspects of Hispanic culture that should be considered in the design of preventive interventions. For example, *machismo* is a characteristic that contributes to substance abuse in males while inhibiting substance use in females (Orlandi, 1986). Schilling et al. (1989) contended that interventions can make use of machismo to emphasize the man's responsibility as head of the family. In addition, the family and neighborhood (*barrio*) are particularly powerful social forces for Hispanic-Americans. Indeed, Mata and Jorquez (1989) concluded that Mexican-American IV drug users continue to rely on social support networks for obtaining drugs and avoiding arrest. As suggested previously for African-Americans, interventions should be delivered through these social systems in the community rather than through formal institutions.

Behavioral Changes in Drug Injection Among IV Drug Users

Several reviews formulated by Des Jarlais and Friedman (Barker et al., 1989; Des Jarlais & Friedman, 1987a, 1988) have documented changes in drug-using behavior among IV drug users since the beginning of the AIDS epidemic. Reviewed studies, however, often have not been published in professional journals, and, consequently, the integrity of their findings has not been submitted to full peer review. With this caveat in mind, the reviewers concluded that IV drug users are usually quite capable of changing their behavior in response to the epidemic. Such changes were reported as early as 1984 among samples of IV drug users in treatment, as well as among those not in treatment; concomitantly, there was much demand for sterile injection equipment on the illicit market (Des Jarlais, Friedman, & Hopkins, 1985). To some extent, these changes in behavior were independent of formal educational and outreach efforts.

Educational and outreach programs that provide convenient methods for behavior change also have had positive effects on the risk-prevention practices of IV drug users, though such conclusions are not based on controlled outcome studies. Ex-addicts have been used successfully to educate IV drug users on appropriate procedures for the decontamination of drug injection equipment (Jackson & Rotkiewicz, 1987). Moreover, upon receiving such education, many of the IV drug users entered treatment programs to reduce the risk of AIDS. Similarly, bleach-distribution programs (e.g., Chaisson, Moss, Onishi, Osmond, & Carlson, 1987) and syringe exchange programs (e.g., van den Hoek, Coutinho, van Zadelhoff, van Haas-Trecht, & Goudsmit, 1988) have evoked behavior change among many IV drug users. Contrary to some predictions, such programs did not lead to an increase in IV drug users or to a decrease in the numbers of IV drug users entering treatment (Barker et al., 1989). In fact, Des Jarlais, Friedman, and colleagues concluded that the implementation of "safer" injection programs may actually decrease rates of injection among IV drug users.

Reviewers (e.g., Barker et al., 1989; Des Jarlais & Friedman, 1987a; 1988) also concluded that there is wide variation in risk-reduction behaviors among IV drug users. For example, new norms against sharing drug injection are strongest among experienced drug users and weakest among those new to the IV drug-using subculture (i.e., adolescents and young adults). In addition, many IV drug users who knew about modes of preventing the transmission of HIV continued to share their equipment and to clean the equipment in ways that would not kill the virus (Flynn et al., 1987). Neaigus et al. (1990) found that the strongest predictors of stopping high-risk drug behavior following an outreach intervention in a sample of IV drug users were low injection frequency at intake and participation in a drug treatment program. Thus those IV drug users at greatest risk for acquiring HIV were least likely to change their high-risk behavior following educational efforts. Clearly, there is a sizable minority of IV drug users, many of whom are young, who continue behaviors that place themselves and others at risk for AIDS.

Changes in Sexual Behavior Among IV Drug Users

IV drug users have engaged in less risk reduction for their sexual behavior than for their drug injection behavior. For example, Ingold and Ingold (1989) reported that the purchase of condoms was uncommon (only 25% of respondents reported such a purchase) and irregular among samples of street addicts and addicts in treatment, even though the respondents were well aware that condom use offered the only effective protection against sexual transmission of HIV. Interestingly, HIV-negative IV drug users reported that they reduced the risk of sexual transmission by avoiding sexual relations with other addicts or by maintaining relations with only a single partner. HIV-positive respondents, on the other hand, indicated that they avoided sexual contact out of a sense of responsibility. If their sexual partner was also HIV-positive, however, then the use of condoms to protect against HIV transmission was irrelevant.

Barker et al. (1989) reviewed eight presentations at the Fourth International AIDS Conference that were related to sexual transmission among IV drug users and concluded that there was minimal use of condoms to reduce sexual transmission of the disease (i.e., only 25% of respondents reported condom use). Likewise, Neaigus et al. (1990), in an uncontrolled experiment, found that participation in an outreach program was linked with a decline in the percentage of IV drug users who engaged in high-risk sexual behavior, but that 59% of respondents still engaged in unprotected sex. Barker et al. (1989) suggested several possible reasons why IV drug users have resisted changing their sexual behaviors. One reason is that perhaps IV drug users fear the introduction of condom use would jeopardize the stability of their interpersonal relationship. Des Jarlais and Friedman (1988) suggested that it is much easier to introduce condom use into casual sexual relationships than into existing emotional relationships. It is also likely that IV drug users have not changed their sexual behavior for the same reasons that members of the general population have not changed their sexual behavior. In any case, the general lack of sexual precautions among IV drug users is certainly a major contributor to the spread of the disease among heterosexuals.

Summary and Conclusions

Transmission of HIV associated with IV drug use has accounted for the majority of AIDS cases among heterosexuals, minorities, and young children. IV drug use is a social activity, and it is likely that the causes of IV drug use in adolescents are multidimensional in nature. Given this condition, interventions should be multifaceted, attending to the broader social ecology of adolescent substance abuse. Evidence suggests that IV drug use is linked with high rates of unsafe sexual activities, and that women IV drug users have several significant barriers to the practice of safe sex. Moreover, IV drug use is disproportionately prevalent among African-Americans and Hispanic-Americans; several cultural factors pertinent to the design of interventions were described. Finally, since the beginning of the AIDS epidemic, there is evidence that IV drug users have changed their drug-using behavior in ways that decrease the spread of HIV, but changes in the unsafe sexual practices of IV drug users are less apparent. Risk reduction among adolescent IV drug users is less evident than among their more experienced counterparts.

SIX

Prevention and Interventions

Prevention

The State of Research and Practice

Investment and training. In the absence of a cure for AIDS, hope for slowing the spread of the epidemic lies primarily in prevention. At least until a vaccine is developed, prevention of AIDS necessarily means diminution of risky behavior and maintenance of safe behavior. Surprisingly little—one might say, appallingly little—investment has been made in prevention of AIDS. Such efforts consume only $1 out of every $2,000 spent by the federal government on health care (Bailey, 1991).

The inattention to prevention is not simply a manifestation of government action; the behavioral sciences also have failed to provide a major focus on prevention. For example, graduate training programs in psychology have shown little interest in educating psychologists to do such work. In late 1987, a survey (Campos, Brasfield, & Kelly, 1989) of all clinical and counseling psychology programs approved by the American Psychological Association (APA) showed that three fourths provided no training at all on AIDS, with courses on AIDS provided in only 2 out of 117 programs. The majority offered no training at all (not even a colloquium) on human sexuality, and almost as many (42% in each case) gave no attention to drug abuse or primary prevention. A parallel survey (also conducted by Campos et al., 1989) of all APA-approved predoctoral internship programs showed that two thirds offered no training in primary prevention or community psychology, and half provided no instruction on human sexuality. Only two internships offered a rotation on AIDS-related services.

Given the paucity of training on children's issues in clinical psychology programs (see, e.g., Magrab & Wohlford, 1990), it is likely that training specifically on prevention of pediatric and adolescent AIDS is virtually nonexistent. The situation is apt to be even worse in disciplines with less history of involvement with developmental and community issues.

Adolescents. Nonetheless, the importance of development of AIDS prevention programs for adolescents cannot be denied. As we noted in Chapter 2, knowledge about age of diagnosis of AIDS and the disease's typical incubation period strongly suggests that HIV infection often occurs at that point in development. More specifically, adolescence is the developmental phase in which initiation into risky drug use or sexual activity typically occurs (if unsafe practices are begun at all); therefore, it probably is the most critical phase for prevention.

As a panel of the National Academy of Sciences (Miller, Turner, & Moses, 1990) has concluded, though, research on preventive interventions, especially among subpopulations at particular risk (e.g., gay youth), is especially lacking for adolescents.

> Owing to the lack of adequate scientific evidence, the committee was able to describe with relative confidence the various patterns of adolescent behavior that place young people at risk of acquiring or transmitting HIV, [but] there is much less certainty about the types of programs that can help adolescents modify those risky behaviors to avoid infection. (p. 202)

The lack of prevention research and the paucity of basic research (e.g., studies of behavior epidemiology) relevant to planning prevention programs directed at adolescents are the result in part of the thorny ethical and legal problems of research on that population, a topic that will be discussed in detail in Chapter 7. Political arguments about the acceptability of discussion of sexual activity and drug use among adolescents may be even more powerful factors in the suppression of such research. As the National Academy of Sciences panel concluded, though, the drawing of moral lines with regard to discussable topics is shortsighted as a practical matter when adult norms about premarital sexual relations are strikingly diverse and most people in the current age cohort become sexually active before age 20 (Miller et al., 1990).

The same factors that have retarded the development of knowledge about AIDS prevention in adolescence have deterred development of programs reasonably likely to be effective. For the most part, the programs now available are school based and educational in form. A study of school-based AIDS education by the General Accounting Office (GAO; Nadel, 1990) found programs in two thirds of American school districts. Unfortunately, though, the prevalence of such educational programs was found to drop off markedly in the 11th and 12th grades (15% coverage), when sexual activity among school-age youth is most likely. Moreover, authorities in two thirds of the districts offering AIDS education reported that their teachers receive no more than 10 hours of training on the subject; one fifth of the teachers received no training at all.

Although the major funder of such programs, the Division of Adolescent and School Health (DASH) of the Centers for Disease Control, expects school districts to provide AIDS education to youths not in school (a group particularly at risk), the GAO (Nadel, 1990) found, unsurprisingly, that such programs are quite small (about 5% of the funds awarded to schools). Six national organizations do have grants to provide AIDS education to out-of-school youths, but these receive only about 5% of total DASH funds for AIDS education.

Principles of Prevention

The ineffectiveness of purely educational approaches. The focus on distribution of factual knowledge about AIDS to low-risk youths (without concomitant emphases on skill deficits and motivational factors) is relatively safe politically, and delivery of school-based AIDS education is relatively easy and inexpensive. The prevalence of such an approach probably is also the product of an erroneous belief: that knowledge by itself will result in less risky behavior. Research generally does not support the assumption that youths engage in risky behavior because they are unaware of the risk. As noted in Chapter

3, although adolescents often believe safe situations also to be risky, they typically are aware of the transmission of HIV through sexual activity and intravenous drug use. Moreover, research on drug education (see Rhodes & Jason, 1988) and sex education for pregnancy prevention (see Hayes, 1987) commonly shows weak effects, if any, on behavior.

Perhaps most fundamentally, the underlying assumption that rational people will not engage in risky behavior if they are informed fully about the risk probably is erroneous. Gardner and Herman (1990) have argued persuasively that risky behavior by adolescents often is explicable by an economic rational-choice model. If one perceives few long-term opportunities, behavior in pursuit of immediate pleasure or gain, even in the face of potentially deadly long-term consequences, is rational, especially if the means of minimization of risk (e.g., use of condoms) are perceived as aversive.

Regardless, it is unreasonable to believe that knowledge will result in behavior change if the audience lacks the skills to use the knowledge, or (as suggested by Gardner and Herman, 1990) if it lacks motivation to acquire or use such skills. This principle was demonstrated to one of us, anecdotally, when he conducted a focus group of student leaders in preparation for an AIDS prevention program for university undergraduates. All of the participants were aware of the nature and benefits of guidelines for safer sex. All, however, also were skeptical about the implementation of the guidelines. In particular, students said that women would be reluctant to bring up the subject of condom use because they feared being perceived as expert on sex and, accordingly, as "loose." Male students also were described as uncomfortable with initiation of discussion of condom use because of fears that their female partners would infer that the men believed them to be promiscuous if the men initiated the discussion.

A subsequent large-scale study on the same campus (Greenwald, Melton, & Nellis, 1991) showed that communication problems do interfere with safer approaches to sexual behavior of college students. Gender roles were also confirmed to be important, although the survey data suggested some dynamics in addition to those identified in the focus group. Notably, men tended to underestimate their own risk, perhaps because of the need to view themselves as "supermen" impervious to harm.

Students, especially women, generally perceived risk as something that others had. The more distant that a comparison was (e.g., you vs. your most likely sexual partner, the average student at this university, the average person in this state, or the average person in the country, in order of increasing distance), the more risk students perceived of AIDS and sexually transmitted diseases (STDs) in general.

In general, peer norms were identified by Melton et al. as important in determining students' sexual behavior. For example, the focus group differentiated norms on campus from those at beach resorts over spring break. Each year, the rate of diagnosis of STDs did rise sharply at the campus studied during the period immediately following spring break. In casual sexual relationships, the motivation for care is apt not to be the same as in continuing relationships.

Studies of IV drug use present similar lessons, in regard both to the critical significance of prevention in adolescence and the psychosocial factors that must be addressed if prevention programs are to be effective. Virtually all IV drug users report having shared needles at least once: the first time that they injected drugs, typically during adolescence (Des Jarlais & Friedman, 1988). Although drug use is multidetermined, its social context is perhaps most important. Peer influences are strong in determining not only whether drug use occurs, but also what the kind of drug and the method of administration will be when it does occur (Turner, Miller, & Moses, 1989).

General principles. Although research on AIDS prevention among adolescents is scant, there is remarkable consistency among commentators about the probable characteristics of successful programs. Such analyses are based on knowledge of (a) the characteristics of successful efforts among adult gay men and IV drug users and (b) the cognitive and social impediments to contraception among teenagers. The National Academy of Sciences panel has stated succinctly the lessons of that work in regard to necessary components of behavior change:

> The committee recommends that, to the extent possible, community-level interventions to prevent the spread of HIV infection address simultaneously information, motivational factors, skills, prevailing norms, and methods for diffusing innovation. (Turner et al., 1989, p. 294)[1]

Summarizing outcome research on prevention among IV drug users, Des Jarlais and Friedman (1988) reached several general conclusions about effective AIDS prevention aimed at that population.

They concurred that basic information is needed, but that information alone is not sufficient to change behavior. They also emphasized the difficulty of successful prevention, in that alteration in risky but rewarding behavior requires sustained reinforcement for such changes if relapse is to be avoided.

Focusing on adolescent prevention programs in particular, Gardner (1991) has argued that prevention efforts must be early, persistent (i.e., using multiple channels), comprehensive (i.e., addressing risk taking in general), inclusive of social skills training, and responsive to the special needs of adolescents already engaging in high-risk behavior. In congressional testimony, Gardner (1991) has identified several policy problems that also must be addressed if such programs are to become widely available:

1. Little is known about adolescent sexual practices or what they mean to youths. *Development of effective, theory-based interventions requires support for basic research on adolescent behavior, and sexual behavior in particular.*

2. Although we should design interventions for young adolescents and preadolescents that will delay the initiation of adult behaviors like alcohol use and sexual intercourse, it is futile and dangerous to deny that the great majority of adolescents are sexually active by the end of high school. *We must face the responsibility of teaching the youths that if they are sexually active, they must protect themselves with condoms.*

3. The adolescents at greatest risk—gay adolescents; runaways; and underclass, delinquent youths—are stigmatized, alienated, and difficult to reach through traditional school or public health interventions. *There must be expanded funding for innovative, research-based programs to deliver prevention services to these groups.* (pp. 7-8)

Peer group strategies. Des Jarlais and Friedman (1988) suggested one mechanism for maintaining behavior change that may have particular relevance to adolescents: intervention to reform peer norms. A focus on peer norms (e.g., group-level interventions) is important in part because of the covariation among sexual activity, substance abuse, and delinquent behavior in youth subcultures that thrive on risky, thrill-seeking behavior (see Osgood & Wilson, 1989). Even among adolescents who generally conform to norms of mainstream culture, norms for developmentally significant steps (e.g., initiation into sexual activity) may be based primarily in the peer culture, as already noted.

Moreover, adoption of safe practices is apt to be facilitated by an affirmative identity (e.g., as a gay youth; as a sexually mature youth) that legitimates planned sexual behavior (see Fisher, 1988) and fosters unexploitive relationships (see Remafedi, 1987b). As has been demonstrated in AIDS prevention among gay men, peer group interventions thus have multiple potential benefits: adoption of new norms, facilitation of planned personal behavior, and enhancement of personal self-esteem through the esteem of others (Joseph et al., 1987). All of these are potential elements in reinforcement of sustained behavior change.

It is noteworthy that the same general principle has been found to apply to AIDS prevention among IV drug users, despite the fact that illegal drug use is associated with antisocial and impulsive behavior. Because needle sharing is largely a part of initiation into IV drug use, development of norms within the established drug culture for safer drug use has proven to be easier to accomplish than many predicted. Stabilization of the incidence of new cases of HIV infection among IV drug users in some locales is, as the National Academy of Sciences panel has noted, "evidence of a capacity and willingness to change risk-associated behaviors in a population that has been characterized in the past as uncooperative and self-destructive" (Turner et al., 1989, p. 214).

In that regard, a focus on street work (e.g., use of ex-addicts as neighborhood AIDS educators) designed to teach safer injection practices is complementary to efforts to reduce drug use. AIDS prevention programs have resulted in increased demand for sterile needles (and a concomitant black market when syringe exchanges are illegal) as well as increased demand for treatment (Des Jarlais & Friedman, 1987b, 1988). This relationship may be the product of increased sense of personal control—and peer support for such an accomplishment—when care has been taken to minimize the risk associated with drug taking.

Some Caveats

Despite the bleak picture painted at the beginning of this chapter, accomplishments in prevention of AIDS have been greater than any other behavior-change campaign within a comparable period of time. Behavior change among IV drug users has been more pronounced than most experts and the general public may have expected, but it has been even more striking among gay men (see Stall, Coates, & Hoff, 1988). That some change in norms about sexual behavior has occurred as a product of the AIDS epidemic is a testament to the intensity and the comprehensiveness of some prevention efforts, especially those generated within the gay community. Nonetheless, the level of behavior change that has occurred is far short of that needed to stem the epidemic, and the task ahead is formidable.

The difficulty in alteration of sexual behavior should not be underestimated. Not only must planning and self-control overtake the pleasure and passion of the "heat of the moment" in lovemaking, but couples must have substantial skill in communication about sensitive matters and mastery of gender-role expectations that may interfere with such communication. The remaining elements of the decision whether to use safer-sex methods are by themselves quite complex:

> Additional psychological obstacles to effective use of contraception may stand in the way, even when an adolescent is knowledgeable about contraception and motivated to use it. Use of contraception requires mastery of a variety of psychological challenges: identification of oneself as sexually active (a fact that, when based on very infrequent intercourse, may be easy to deny), acceptance of erotic feelings and sexuality itself (an attitude that is particularly relevant to use of condoms because of the necessity of genital manipulation), overcoming expectations of negative reactions of the druggist in order to purchase contraceptives, overcoming fear that one will be perceived as "easy" or "experienced" because of preparation for intercourse, reversal of usual gender roles in regard to responsibility for contraception, and interruption of the "spontaneity" of romantic lovemaking. Such factors must be taken into account in teaching decision-making skills or altering public attitudes if education about use of condoms is to be effective. (Melton, 1988a, p. 406)

The difficulty in achieving sustained change in sexual behavior is illustrated by the fact that change in needle-sharing behavior has proven to be easier than change in IV drug users' sexual behavior (Lewis, Das, Hoppner, & Jencks, 1991). Analogously, even drug use itself may be implicated in HIV infections in some populations more often because of its association with unsafe sex than because of the drug use itself. For example, because use of cocaine often leads to high-risk sexual behavior, it is a greater factor in AIDS among adolescents than is intravenous drug use (Miller et al., 1990).

Prevention programs must take into account individual differences in values and behaviors. Although the principles outlined in this chapter appear to be widely generalizable, prevention planners still need to take into account the particular needs and responses of special populations of adolescents. Such special populations do not necessarily correspond to groups living outside the mainstream of the broader society. For example, athletes are a little-targeted group that may be at particular risk in some localities, because athletes are especially likely to abuse anabolic steroids intravenously (see Nemechek, 1991).

Perhaps more obviously, the frequency of risk-taking behavior varies enormously, and prevention strategies should be altered accordingly. Although most adolescents become sexually active before leaving their teenage years, the modal reported frequency of intercourse among sexually active teenage girls is zero (Hayes, 1987). For such youth, a major problem of prevention is to induce a perception of oneself as sexually active so that appropriate planning has been made for the instances in which intercourse does take place.

By contrast, about 15% of sexually active youth are "sexual adventurers," who have multiple partners without emotional relationships (Sorensen, 1973). Such youth typically engage in diverse impulsive behavior (perhaps including drug use), and they may not be amenable to prevention through conventional avenues (e.g., school-based programs). To be effective, prevention programs aimed at such youth must go where the youth themselves are and adapt to the sometimes chaotic life-styles that they pursue. Similar issues apply to AIDS education for runaway and "throwaway" youths (Rotheram-Borus, Koopman, Haignere, & Davies, 1991).

To maximize effectiveness, prevention programs should provide unambiguous messages. Mixed messages about safer sex and drug use yield framing effects that result in greater risky behavior. For example, Yale undergraduates were asked, "Should the government allow this condom to be advertised and sold as an effective method for preventing the spread of AIDS?" When told that the condom was 95% effective, about 90% answered positively. On the other hand, when the condom was described as having a 5% failure rate, only 42% agreed

(Dawes, 1988). There is reason to believe that results at least as pronounced would be obtained if high school students were surveyed in a similar manner.

Prevention programs must overcome cognitive unavailability. Perhaps the most difficult problem of AIDS prevention in adolescence is that, because of the lengthy latency of symptoms typical in HIV infection, adolescents are unlikely to know anyone their own age who has AIDS (even though some of their peers may be infected). Studies of adult gay men have shown that personal knowledge of someone who has AIDS facilitates behavior change (McKusick, Horstman, & Coates, 1985). Accordingly, AIDS education programs directed at adolescents must increase the salience of risk of fatal illness a decade later.

Public policy should make safer behavior as easy to accomplish as possible. The psychological and fiscal costs of use of condoms and sterile syringes must be reduced for sexually active and drug-using youth. Embarrassment and high cost can exact a high price: failure to take preventive measures. Because adolescents have relatively little experience in negotiating the marketplace, they are deterred easily by apparent obstacles. Moreover, because they typically have quite limited finances, their demand for products is highly susceptible to variations in price (see, e.g., Lewitt, Coate, & Grossman, 1981). Therefore, the place of distribution of condoms, for example, should be easily accessible, and the price should be minimal or zero.

For widespread preventive effects, broad changes in social policy may be necessary. Ultimately, a reduction of the stigma attached to AIDS (see Herek & Glunt, 1988) may be necessary if prevention is to be effective. Such stigma enhances the perception that risk of AIDS is something to which someone else is subject. Even more fundamental social change also may be necessary: The literature on contraception by adolescents shows that the perception of a future in which one can exercise personal control and achieve upward mobility is an important determinant of sexually responsible behavior (Hayes, 1987). Widespread achievement of such a view may require objective changes in the opportunities available to disadvantaged youth. At a minimum, it demands participation by youth themselves in the design of preventive efforts.

Similar problems apply to prevention of pediatric AIDS. The nature of the social change that is needed is clear when one acknowledges that the principal transmitters of pediatric AIDS are women who are poor, who have ethnic minority background, and who are involved in relationships in which they are often exploited and abused.

For both adolescent and pediatric AIDS, social change (including appropriations to expand treatment programs and necessary legal reforms to permit consent to treatment by youths themselves) also is needed to make treatment easily available for adolescents and young adults who are IV drug users or often are engaged in other risky behavior. In that regard, treatment of drug dependence and conduct disorders can be conceptualized as prevention of AIDS.

Medical Interventions

Although a detailed description of clinical pharmacology is beyond the scope of this volume, a basic understanding of AIDS treatment efforts is essential for individuals who are likely to work with children and families living with AIDS. Therefore, we present a brief overview of currently used pharmacological agents and their reported effectiveness in treating HIV infection and AIDS in children and adolescents. Compliance problems and impediments to medical treatment are also discussed.

Medical Treatments for HIV and AIDS in Children and Adolescents

Urgency has characterized the efforts to develop effective treatments for pediatric AIDS. Enhancing the quality and duration of life for children with HIV infection or AIDS is an essential therapeutic endeavor. Prior to the discovery and characterization of HIV as the etiologic agent of AIDS, treatment consisted primarily of supportive care through the management of secondary infections. Although opportunistic infections continue to be one focus of medical attention, today's therapeutic efforts are aimed also at developing pharmacological interventions to control or eliminate HIV replication (Haseltine, 1989; Jeffries, 1989). Directing clinical research at the underlying cause of AIDS is critical because initiation of treatment early in the HIV life cycle (i.e., while the child is asymptomatic) may preserve normal immunological and neurological functioning, two symptoms associated with pediatric AIDS that are directly related to viral replication, and delay or prevent disease progression (Balis & Poplack, 1991).

Balis and Poplack (1991) have highlighted several problems concerning the development and use of new pharmacologic therapies. First, pharmacologic agents presently under development show little promise for total eradication of latent HIV infection without destroying many other critical cellular structures. Consequently, lifelong pharmacotherapy is likely; it is also difficult to manufacture antiretroviral agents that are inexpensive, easily administered, and without long-term toxicities or side effects. Second, developing an agent that prevents transmission of the virus is a problem. Clearly, inhibiting viral excretion and transmission of HIV is an important milestone in containing the AIDS pandemic and should be a principal focus of drug development. Third, a pharmacologic agent must be able to penetrate the blood-brain barrier in order to control HIV infection in the central nervous system (CNS). Fourth, as noted previously, it seems imperative that drug therapy begin during the early phase of HIV infection. By initiating treatment while the individual is asymptomatic, complications associated with managing opportunistic infections during the later phases of infection may be avoided. Finally, newborns and infants pose a particular problem for drug development. Their rapid changes in body composition and organ function present a unique and difficult treatment challenge.

Once a new pharmacologic agent has been developed, clinical trials are performed by experienced investigators under the supervision of the Federal Drug Administration (FDA). Clinical trials must progress successfully through three phases prior to receiving approval for routine administration to humans. Phase I involves the administration of the new agent to individuals who have not responded to conventional therapy. The primary goals of this phase are to determine the maximum tolerated dose (MTD) of the new agent and its toxicities or side effects. Phase II involves delineating the degree of clinical effect inherent in the agent. For instance, investigators during this phase may examine the efficacy of the agent with respect to its impact on the number of opportunistic infections, CD4:CD8 ratio, and neuropsychological functioning. During Phase III, an empirical evaluation of the new agent is conducted. Specifically, the new agent may be compared or used in combination with conventional therapy.

As one might expect, the criteria for using newly developed pharmacologic agents in clinical trials with children are quite stringent. Children generally cannot be enrolled in clinical trials until Phase I with adults has established a maximum tolerated dose. Consequently, clinical trials with children often lag 1 to 2 years behind those for adults. Delaying clinical trials for children until the completion of Phase I trials for adults has generated considerable public outcry, which may soon lead to modification of this policy (Novello, Wise, Willoughby, & Pizzo, 1989). Moreover, FDA criteria for final drug approval seem easier to meet for adults than for children. For instance, azidothymidine (AZT) was approved rather quickly for use with adults, but encountered numerous delays in gaining approval for its use with children. Approximately 34 centers have conducted or presently are conducting pediatric clinical trials as part of the AIDS Clinical Trials Group (ACTG), sponsored by the National Institute of Allergy and Infectious Disease (NIAID); the majority of these trials are presently in Phase I or Phase II. The number of pediatric clinical trials is expected to increase soon as the ACTG and the National Institute of Child Health and Development (NICHD) merge their clinical trial efforts.

Several reverse transcriptase inhibitors have been developed and are being evaluated in clinical trials. AZT (which is also known as zidovudine) was the first antiretroviral agent approved by the FDA for treating AIDS in adults (Fischl et al., 1990; Volberding et al., 1990). In October 1987, it received FDA approval for use with children over 12 years of age who had symptomatic HIV infection. In 1989, the FDA approved the use of AZT for children under 13 years of age, and in early 1990, it was licensed for use with all children. Presently, AZT is being evaluated as a therapeutic agent in symptomatic and asymptomatic infants, children, and HIV-infected women during their third trimester of pregnancy. It now serves as the prototype for the development of other antiretroviral agents (e.g., dideoxycytidine, or ddC; dideoxyinosine, or ddI). Other agents that inhibit the attachment of HIV to receptor sites (e.g., recombinant CD4, immunoglobulins) are also being evaluated (Pizzo & Wilfert, 1991).

Pizzo and Wilfert (1991) provide an excellent review of the findings from clinical trials with children using dideoxynucleosides. Overall, both intravenous and oral AZT administration have yielded positive results in Phase I trials. In one study evaluating continuous infusion of AZT via Hickman-Broviac catheter, Pizzo et al. (1988) found that all 13 children with documented neurodevelopmental abnormalities demonstrated improvement in HIV encephalopathy symptoms within 1 to 3 weeks after beginning AZT treatment. Neuro-developmental improvements consisted of reacquisition of lost developmental milestones (e.g., speech, walking, other motor activities) as well as general improvement in affect and activity.

Moreover, significant improvements in cognitive functioning were demonstrated after only 6 months of continuous-infusion AZT. Using standardized measures of intelligence (e.g., Wechsler Intelligence Scale for Children—Revised, McCarthy Scales of Children's Abilities, and Bayley Scales of Infant Development), the authors demonstrated an improvement in IQ scores of 1 standard deviation at 6-month follow-up in children with pre-AZT neurodevelopmental abnormalities. It is noteworthy that those children who initially appeared free of neurodevelopmental abnormalities prior to receiving AZT demonstrated equally substantial improvements in IQ scores, perhaps suggesting the possibility that these children manifested subclinical cognitive impairment not detected prior to treatment. A recent follow-up study revealed that gains in intellectual functioning were maintained after 12 months of AZT therapy, and it documented similar improvements in adaptive behavior over time (Brouwers et al., 1990). Although these findings are marred by methodological limitations (e.g., small *n*, IQ scores from different tests, no randomization, few subjects with pre-HIV data), they demonstrate the potential neurodevelopmental benefit of AZT therapy in children.

Other researchers have found that children with AIDS show some early signs of improvement with AZT treatment, but long-term gains after 1 year of receiving AZT have not been demonstrated (Pizzo & Wilfert, 1991). In fact, a significant percentage of children with AIDS develop intolerance or become refractory to AZT treatment, and others develop bone marrow toxicity necessitating dose reductions or discontinuation of AZT. Early studies of dideoxycytidine (ddC) and dideoxyinosine (ddI) in symptomatic children have found them to be well tolerated and not associated with bone marrow suppression (see review by Pizzo & Wilfert, 1991). Recombinant CD4 (rCD4), which inhibits the attachment of viral cells to receptor sites, has demonstrated some effectiveness in adults (Schooley et al., 1990) but has not been evaluated as a treatment for HIV infection in children. There is hope that rCD4 can be used to block transplacental transmission of HIV from mother to fetus.

Medical management of adolescents with HIV infection presents unique concerns. Clearly, changes in body composition during adolescence, including increased body fat among females and muscle mass among males, may have direct effects on drug dose, dose interval, toxicity, and effectiveness (Futterman & Hein, 1991; Hein, 1987b). Furthermore, tobacco, alcohol, or illicit drug use may affect drug metabolism among adolescents. Because adolescents were not considered part of the Pediatric Clinical Trials Group until 1989, the effectiveness of various pharmacological agents has yet to be evaluated.

The majority of AZT studies have involved children with vertically transmitted HIV; only a few have included protocols for children with hemophilia (e.g., Lusher & Warrier, 1991). The number of HIV-infected children and adolescents with hemophilia participating in clinical trials is expected to increase, however, because the 10 hemophilia regional coordinating centers have been integrated into the ACTG. Offering AZT to adolescents with hemophilia and asymptomatic HIV infection appears to be standard medical procedure. Without additional data, though, regarding the efficacy of AZT in younger children with hemophilia, Lusher and Warrier (1991) reported that most physicians are restricting AZT use in children under 12 years of age to those who are symptomatic.

Compliance Problems and Impediments
to Providing Care

Multiple daily administrations of antiretroviral agents, frequent medical appointments, repeated physical examinations, and careful attention to caloric intake suggest that the medical regimen for children and adolescents with HIV infection or AIDS may be complex and time-consuming. Given the other problems faced by an HIV-infected and/or IV drug-using parent of a young child, or a homeless IV drug-using adolescent, compliance with the prescribed medical regimen may be especially problematic. For some adolescents with HIV infection and young mothers of HIV-infected children, compliance with medical treatment may be a less immediate need than food, shelter, and/or illicit drugs.

Furthermore, data now suggest that antiretroviral agents must be administered orally for prolonged periods of time. Although there is a strawberry-flavored syrup form of AZT for young children, we presently do not have data on the rate of noncompliance in this population of children. Extrapolating from research on children with other medical conditions requiring frequent administrations of medications, we can expect moderately high rates of noncompliance and partial compliance (La Greca, 1988).

Pizzo (1990) outlined several other problems in providing medical care to children and adolescents with HIV infection or AIDS. For instance, although the prevailing policy is to enroll as many children as possible in clinical trials, many parents and guardians of HIV-infected children either are not enrolling their children and wards in research protocols or are withdrawing from studies prematurely. Furthermore, there is a need for increased cooperation among medical specialties (e.g., pediatrics, obstetrics, adolescent medicine) with a special focus on treating children with AIDS. Pizzo (1990) also notes that family dynamics, including the possibility that more than one family member has AIDS, may affect adherence behaviors and may make medical treatment especially difficult.

Psychosocial Considerations/Interventions

Data concerning the rising incidence of pediatric AIDS and its treatment highlight an emergent need to examine variables affecting the psychosocial adaptation of children with AIDS and their families. It has been suggested that children with HIV infection or AIDS and their families may be at increased risk for psychosocial problems (e.g., Olson, Huszti, Mason, & Seibert, 1989; Wiener & Septimus, 1991). Uncertain medical prognosis, a complex medical regimen, heightened and recurrent stress, anticipatory grief, disruption in family activities, increase in caretaker burden, and social stigmatization and isolation secondary to public fears and misperceptions could potentially increase the psychological vulnerability of these children and their families. For example, Seibert, Garcia, Kaplan, and Septimus (1989) reported that primary caregivers of children with HIV infection or AIDS commonly experience feelings of anxiety, depression, guilt, and grief, as well as concerns regarding their own physical health status, death, and parenting competence. Primary caregivers also expressed concerns about their child's attachment difficulties, poor health status, and developmental aberrations. The fact that many of these families have extremely limited financial resources, histories of excessive drug use, and more than one chronically ill member may foreshadow additional problems in psychosocial adaptation. Despite the perceived psychological risk of children with AIDS and their families, though, it is important to remember that much of what has been written about the psychosocial sequelae of pediatric AIDS is anecdotal and descriptive; well-controlled, systematic investigations in this area are lacking, and definitive statements regarding the psychosocial functioning of children with AIDS and their families are premature.

Several authors have argued for a multisystemic or social-ecological approach to treating chronically ill children and their families (Henggeler & Borduin, 1990; Kazak, 1989). Indeed, in light of the social-ecological complexities of pediatric AIDS, health professionals working with children with AIDS must assess, and consider within the context of intervention, the numerous individual, familial, and extrafamilial variables that potentially can affect outcome. Garmezy (1987), for instance, noted that predicting a child's psychosocial vulnerability requires knowledge about the child's disposition, the supportiveness of the family environment, and the quality of the social support system. Certainly, in pediatric AIDS, the latter two dimensions (family and social support) may be cause for great concern, because parents themselves may be disabled by AIDS, and the stigmatization and fears surrounding the AIDS pandemic may affect how communities respond to affected children and their families (Kazak, 1989).

As the treatment of pediatric AIDS becomes increasingly multisystemic and interdisciplinary, pediatric psychologists are being asked to play an important role in terms of assessment, intervention, and research. The pediatric psychology consultation-liaison service at the University of Florida Health Sciences Center provides a model for how pediatric psychologists might be part of an interdisciplinary approach to treating children and adolescents with HIV infection or AIDS and their families. The consultation-liaison service, a subspecialty of the Department of Clinical and Health Psychology, provides diagnostic, consultation, and therapeutic services for ambulatory and hospitalized children and adolescents with acute or chronic illnesses and their families. Pediatric psychologists work collaboratively with various medical teams (e.g., oncology, infectious diseases, cardiology) in providing care to children and adolescents with medical problems, including those with HIV infection or AIDS, and their families. It is essential that the pediatric psychologist have a solid background in general clinical psychology as well as familiarity with various pediatric ailments and their respective treatments. Indeed, the special knowledge and expertise assessing the complex interactions among physical, psychological, and social factors allows the pediatric psychologist to bridge the specialties of psychology and medicine.

Consultations are requested by the child's physician or another member of the medical team, usually in response to concerns regarding the impact of the illness (e.g., HIV infection or AIDS) on the psychosocial functioning of the child or family. In the case of a child with HIV infection or AIDS, concerns regarding psychological adjustment are coupled with questions about the child's cognitive status. In such instances, these individuals are provided with developmental, cognitive, and behavioral evaluations. In addition, psychosocial assessments of the unique strengths and vulnerabilities of the affected individual and family are conducted routinely. Interventions then are designed and implemented to meet the special needs of the individual and/or family (e.g., pain and stress management, grief counseling, supportive psychotherapy, family therapy, peer education).

In some instances, hospitalized children with AIDS or their families are referred to the pediatric psychology consultation-liaison service to assist in managing special problems that affect medical care and physical status. For example, a hospitalized 3-year-old child with AIDS may refuse to eat or take prescribed oral medications. Following a comprehensive assessment of individual, familial, and contextual variables, as well as appropriate consultation with the medical team, a behavior management program might be designed and implemented in collaboration with the child's parents, physician, and nurse. At other times, the pediatric psychologist may serve as a liaison between the patient or family and the health care system to clarify misunderstandings between the family and the medical team or to assist in accessing needed medical or psychological services. Finally, because many patients and families travel great distances for treatment, referrals often are made to appropriate mental health professionals in the patient's home community.

It is essential that health professionals involved in the treatment of children with AIDS and their families possess a basic understanding of the nature of HIV infection and AIDS as well as its concomitant treatment demands on the child and family. Because of the secrecy and social sensitivity that often accompany AIDS, children and family members may quickly form a negative opinion of the health professional who lacks adequate knowledge, who does not understand the complexities and problems of living with AIDS, or who does not demonstrate proper consideration for the social-ecological context in which the child and family are embedded. Indeed, studies have demonstrated that few mental health professionals possess adequate knowledge of pediatric AIDS. Furthermore, even fewer health professionals have had training in assessment and intervention techniques with this population of children (Sheridan, Coates, Chesney, Beck, & Morokoff, 1989). Recognition and remediation of one's knowledge gaps with respect to pediatric AIDS and an appreciation for the social-ecological factors influencing psychosocial adaptation are necessary first steps for those aspiring to provide mental health services to children with HIV infection or AIDS and their families.

Note

1. See also Flora and Thoresen (1988) on application of social learning theory to AIDS prevention and Lewis, Battistich, and Schaps (1990) on school-based prevention programs.

SEVEN

Ethical and Legal Issues

Perhaps never before has a disease, or any particular health condition, raised so many legal and ethical problems that it has become the focus of entire courses in law schools. With life and death hanging in the balance, AIDS presents extraordinary conflicts involving groups often already subjected to social stigma and discrimination. Hundreds of legal cases (including about 200 criminal prosecutions) related to AIDS have been decided in the short but deadly history of the disease (Sherman, 1991b; for a list of cases, see Gostin, 1990a, 1990b).

The issues at stake are so profound that one distinguished legal commentator, Dean Monroe Price (1989) of the Benjamin N. Cardozo School of Law at Yeshiva University, has argued that AIDS may reorder the relation between the individual and the state. He has gone so far as to suggest that the need to provide AIDS education—"suddenly to open windows into the minds and souls of millions—[may] be seen by powerful institutions as a moment for reshaping the American character in its totality, not just as a change to adjust that character to the needs of the moment" (p. 16).

Consensus rarely has emerged from the socially and personally profound, emotionally charged, and intellectually difficult debates that have typified law and policy on AIDS. For example, a recent national survey of state school administrators (Hartwig & Eckland, 1991) showed consensus (defined as two-thirds agreement) on only

99

9 of 25 policy questions related to AIDS and education. Low levels of agreement were found on such questions as whether records of children with HIV infection should be shared with other agencies, whether state health departments should promulgate rules affecting children with HIV infection, whether such children should be referred to special education, and whether they could be removed from school on the basis on their behavior. The items on which there was consensus generally were flag-and-apple-pie statements about the role of the schools (e.g., "It is the duty of school administrators to ensure the health and safety of all children"; "Local school boards should have a policy regarding admission of HIV-positive children").

The "solutions" offered by the general public to problems related to AIDS are equally diverse and sometimes draconian. More than three fourths of the American public favor criminal charges (murder, 50%; assault, 29%) for anyone who spreads the HIV virus, and the majority advocate criminal liability specifically if a child is born disabled as a result of substance abuse during pregnancy (Sherman, 1991a).

Conflicts of Interest

At root, the intensity of the public response to AIDS rests in the fact that the conflicts of interest that are the foci of policy debates are both pervasive and profound. For example, AIDS activists' demands for a level of protection of confidentiality that goes beyond even that which is typical in matters related to health conditions are based on a recognition of the extraordinary personal costs that can result from a breach of confidentiality. Disclosure of individuals' HIV-positive status may subject them to intrusion into the most private aspects of their lives (e.g., their sexual behavior, relationships, and health habits), social stigma as a disease carrier and often as a member of another stigmatized group, and even criminal penalties. Such disclosure also violates the implied or expressed contract between patients and their doctors; a breach of confidentiality is a wrong apart from the harm that it does.

The interests of people with HIV infection coincide to some extent with those of the public as a whole. Recognizing that many individuals who are infected with HIV realistically fear prejudice (and its products) if their serostatus is disclosed, some public health authorities have advocated the application of "superconfidentiality" to personal information (e.g., serostatus) related to AIDS. Their espousal of protection of the privacy of people infected with HIV (as well as those who seek HIV testing but whose serostatus is negative) commonly is based on a belief that such action is in the public interest. Breaches of confidentiality may deter people from seeking diagnosis and treatment; such intrusions on privacy also may disrupt existing therapeutic relationships based on an implicit contract that health professionals will, "above all, do no harm" to their patients. Additional harm to the public health may result directly from failure to maintain such relationships and possibly to sustain behavior change that will minimize the spread of HIV.

At the same time, the passionate—even if not fully informed or realistic—fear that accompanies a disease that is both infectious and deadly leads to a concern with ensuring that the "need to know" is protected at least as much as confidentiality. Sometimes this need is based on objectively sound concerns: a serious risk of infection in a context in which few believe themselves to be at risk (e.g., currently monogamous sexual partners in a low-prevalence area). At other times, such a need derives from a fear of casual contagion that is objectively groundless but psychologically real.

The level of conflicting interests perhaps is illustrated best by recognition of the fact that people with HIV infection often have an interest not only in protection of confidentiality but also in retention of identifiable data (American Psychological Association [APA], 1985/1986; Melton & Gray, 1988). Storage of clinical records obviously permits ongoing health care as advances in treatment even of asymptomatic patients arise. Similarly, retention of identifiable research data makes notification of participants possible when advances in treatment occur or when new studies require participants with particular characteristics. Such studies may result in information that is helpful not only to other people with HIV infection but also to the participants themselves. Retention of data also is necessary for longitudinal research to illuminate the natural history of HIV and thus provide information that may result not only in a better understanding of the disease and new directions for clinical research but in the identification of long-term needs for treatment and economic support and the corollary refinement of public policy. Again, these developments may benefit participants themselves as well as others in a similar situation.

Not only are the interests of people with HIV infection complex and sometimes conflicting, but professionals also sometimes have concerns of their own that may affect their judgment in dilemmas that arise in work related to AIDS. Of course, professionals are not immune from prejudice; this point will be discussed later in this chapter. Moreover, notable work on AIDS may bring tenure, merit pay, patent royalties, and even celebrity status. One of the uglier aspects of the scientific community's response to the AIDS epidemic has been public wrangling (even lawsuits) over credit for advances in knowledge—a spectacle that has resulted in doubt about the validity of claims made by some scientists (see, e.g., Hamilton, 1991) and that has exacerbated skepticism of some AIDS activists about the motives of professionals in science and health care.

The Complication of Complex Interests

Parents and Children

Specialists in child and family policy typically do not face concerns of life-or-death proportions, and they rarely are placed in situations in which they are tempted by fame and fortune. They are accustomed, however, to dealing with intense conflicts of interest among parents, children, and the state that are so complex that it is often difficult to discern when particular interests (including the child's own interest in protection of autonomy and privacy) coincide with the child's best interest (see Melton, 1987; Mnookin & Weisberg, 1989).

Given the nature of the debates that surround both AIDS policy and child and family policy, it is unsurprising that ethical and legal issues pertaining to children, adolescents, and families have presented some of the most intractable and emotionally charged problems in the AIDS epidemic. Such issues are complicated further by some of the developmental peculiarities of HIV. For example, a test for HIV antibodies in the blood of neonates is a reliable indicator of the serostatus of the mother but not the infant. Accordingly, mandatory HIV testing of newborns is a direct intrusion not only on parental autonomy (an interest that has given way to public health and child-protection concerns in relation to some other pediatric illnesses) but also on the mother's personal privacy.

Even if the state would not otherwise force itself between parents and a child, it may be compelled to do so when a mother's judgment may be clouded by the realities of her own condition (including possible neurological impairment) as well as by the social problems that are likely to have made her vulnerable to HIV infection. At a minimum, the usual assumption of unity of interest of parent and child may reasonably be questioned when the family is overwhelmed with profound social, psychological, economic, and medical needs.[1] Put bluntly, can a drug-addicted, terminally ill mother who long has experienced a chaotic life-style, economic deprivation, and abusive, exploitive relationships, and whose intellect is impaired by emotional disturbance and dementia, be depended upon to protect her child's interests?[2] The debate about state intrusion into the lives of families of children with HIV infection thus can be seen in the light of the broader controversy about the legitimacy of state interference with the rights of substance-abusing parents and pregnant women (see, e.g., *Johnson v. State,* 1991; for an overview of state statutes on commitment of drug-dependent persons and the implications of such statutes for drug-abusing pregnant women, see Garcia & Keilitz, 1991).

Life Expectancy as a Factor

Ethical and legal problems related to pediatric AIDS also are complicated by the fact that it is unclear how a child's diminished life expectancy—which, in fact, is not as brief as even many health care professionals actually involved in the care of children with AIDS believe it to be (Levin, Driscoll, & Fleischman, 1991)[3]—should affect policy and case management. A plausible argument can be made, for example, that children who are nearly certain to die in childhood should be given only whatever care is likely to make their life more comfortable. Heroic health care measures and even education may not improve their quality of life. Health care professionals, in fact, say that they would be less likely to provide necessary surgery for children of women with AIDS than children without such a history (Levin et al., 1991).

It should be noted, though, that such an argument may be based less on concern for the welfare of children with HIV infection than on prejudice. Overtly, it is based on an assumption that the experiences that are valuable to children in general are not so valuable to children with a life-threatening illness—an idea that may have merit in some cases but that also may be a denial of the needs and feelings of a group for whom some may simply not wish to invest resources, whether because of a rather callous cost-benefit analysis or because of a disdain for the group.

In this regard, it is clear that health service providers are not immune from prejudice toward people with AIDS. For example, mental health professionals, especially those without specialized training on AIDS, indicate that they would be less likely to accept for treatment a client with AIDS than one with leukemia (Crawford, Humfleet, Ribordy, Ho, & Vickers, 1991). Physicians who are relatively homophobic also tend to be relatively ignorant about AIDS (Lewis, Freeman, & Corey, 1987). Many physicians, even in high-prevalence areas, say that they would not allow their children to visit the home of a person with AIDS and that they would not attend a party where a person with AIDS was preparing food (Kelly, St. Lawrence, Smith, Hood, & Cook, 1987b).

There also is evidence that the public is ambivalent about provision of special education for children of drug abusers, even when they are not infected with HIV (Murphy-Berman & Sullivan, 1991). Children thus may be penalized because their parents are perceived as undeserving.

Moreover, the "quality of life" argument raises suspicion that its proponents place diminished value on the lives of children with serious disabilities. The debate about provision of resources for children with AIDS reminds one of the analogous furor over the proper allocation of responsibility for decision making in "Baby Doe" cases (a debate in which advocacy organizations for people with disabilities typically line up on the side of lifesaving treatment without regard to a child's other disabilities). As the Baby Doe examples show, though, the question of proper treatment of children with AIDS is not a simple one. This point was illustrated further by a moving series of stories in the *Washington Post* (e.g., Weiser, 1991) about the anguish experienced by the attending physician and nurses, and the foster parents themselves, when a fundamentalist couple refused to permit removal of life supports for their 16-month-old foster child, who was dying of AIDS.

Whatever the ethics of the situation, the shortened life expectancy of children and adolescents with HIV infection makes legal relief easier to obtain when discrimination in provision of services does occur. One of the criteria for obtaining a preliminary injunction is that a delay in reaching a judgment will result in irreparable harm—a criterion that on its face is applicable to children with a terminal illness, who literally have little time to wait (*Robertson v. Granite City Community Unit School District No. 9,* 1988).

Who Should Decide?

Adolescents

The determination of the interests at stake in matters pertaining to children and adolescents with HIV infection is directly relevant to the allocation of responsibility for decision making. As we have already noted, the often chaotic lifestyles of parents of children with vertically transmitted HIV infection raise questions in such cases about whether such parents are able to protect their children's interests.

Somewhat different questions often arise in cases of adolescents who have, or who are at risk for, HIV infection. In some of the high-risk groups (e.g., runaway and "throwaway" youth), parents' and their children's interests may indeed be adverse, and the state consequently may have an interest in protection of such teenagers that is sufficiently strong to justify limitations on parental autonomy. Such an interest may be vindicated by either coercive intervention into family life (i.e., use of child-protective jurisdiction, usually through the family court) or state support for youth autonomy (i.e., recognition of a right for teenagers to obtain independently diagnosis, treatment, or counseling related to AIDS).

The state also may grant youths power of consent in recognition of their liberty and privacy interests. Sexuality is viewed consensually as a domain that falls well within a "zone" of privacy. Accordingly, just as abortion and contraception are domains in which the courts have recognized fundamental rights such as that of minors to consent to abortion (although states may limit these rights more than those of adults; see *Hodgson v. Minnesota,* 1990), states may decide on policy grounds (even if a constitutional interest is not recognized) to permit minors to consent independently to HIV testing, treatment, and counseling because of the privacy interests that are at stake.

Some states have adopted statutes explicitly providing such a right to adolescents. For example, California (1988/1990) permits minors who are 12 or older to consent independently to HIV testing, and New Jersey (1989/1991) uses the same age marker for control of records relating to HIV infection. Wisconsin (1989/1990) sets 14 as the age of consent to services related to AIDS. Iowa (1988b/1989) provides all minors with authority to consent to HIV testing, but it requires that they be informed that positive test results will be disclosed to parents. Going further, New York (1988/1991) effectively treats minors as adults for the purpose of consenting to health services related to AIDS; the relevant statute permits independent consent by anyone who has the capacity to consent, "determined without regard to the individual's age."

Even when no specific statutory authority exists for minors' consent to diagnosis and treatment of HIV infection, such a right may apply on other grounds (for general reviews of minors' ability to consent to mental health and physical health services, respectively, see Melton & Ehrenreich, in press; and Wadlington, 1983). Whether by statute or common law, states generally recognize a class of *emancipated* minors who are able to enter into contracts as if they were adults. In some states, the criteria for emancipation are sufficiently broad that they encompass most youths who are living independently, including runaways. Providers should be aware, though, that the standard for emancipation can be quite narrow. For example, Nebraska (1988) recognizes only married minors as emancipated.

Some states also recognize a *mature minor* rule, under which at least older adolescents who are de facto competent are permitted to consent to treatment. Even if such a rule is not applied to all health care decisions, it may be established for particular conditions or forms of treatment. The most widely applicable exception to the general rule that minors are per se incompetent to consent to health care is that all states permit minors to seek diagnosis and treatment of sexually transmitted diseases (STDs). In states in which the health department or the legislature itself defines HIV infection as an STD, adolescents should be able to seek HIV testing and treatment independently. Nonetheless, in the majority of states, no express statutory authority exists for recognition of adolescents' ability to consent to services related to HIV infection, and the scope of any common-law mature minor rule is likely to be ambiguous, because such issues are rarely litigated.

Four caveats are worth mentioning for the benefit of practitioners even in states where explicit authority exists for minors to consent to HIV-related health care. First, the availability of clear legal permission for service providers to treat adolescents does not absolve clinicians from exercising due care. For example, just as it may be argued that clinicians should seek adolescents' consent in states where parental permission is legally sufficient, the converse may also be true. Regardless, HIV-related counseling often will involve "coming-out" issues (Slater, 1988) that require special ethical and clinical sensitivity.

Second, that an adolescent may consent independently to diagnosis and treatment (enterprises that are typically constructed in his or her own interest) does not necessarily imply a right to consent independently to research, a matter about which state laws typically are silent (Melton, 1989a). Even though the federal regulations on research provide for minors' consent to research without parental permission when they are able to consent independently to treatment for related health services (Department of Health & Human Services [DHHS], 1991a, §46.402[a]), that section is preempted if state laws are more protective. (For more detailed discussions of research ethics and law related to AIDS, see Gray, 1989; Gray & Melton, 1985.)

Third, permission for youths in general to consent independently, whether to treatment or research, should not be construed necessarily to vest such authority in adolescents who are in the care of the state. Because such youths are believed to be especially vulnerable, review by a third party may be necessary, as in fact is required for research involving state wards (DHHS, 1991a, §46.409).

Fourth, the right to consent *independently* does not necessarily imply a right to consent *confidentially*. The latter right flows from the former only if the former is based on support for autonomy and privacy. It is not necessarily a corollary if the consent law is premised on the need to facilitate access to treatment. Note, for example, that the Iowa (1988b/1989) statute mentioned earlier expressly denies confidentiality against parents to minors who obtain HIV-related services independently.

Pregnant Women

Although adults usually are presumed competent to consent and, therefore, are granted the right to decide for themselves whether to accept treatment or participate in research, questions nonetheless are alive about the rights of pregnant women in matters related to HIV infection.[4] This controversy is derived from the larger issue of the limits of women's control over their own bodies when another life is at stake. Whether the testing is mandatory or voluntary, HIV testing of pregnant women inevitably raises the issue of abortion, as applied to fetuses that are at risk of being born with an HIV infection.

Although favoring freedom in the decisions about whether to obtain HIV testing and/or an abortion, a panel of the American Medical Association (AMA, 1990) framed the problem as an analogue to Baby Doe issues as well as a question of reproductive choice:

> Promoting abortion to achieve public health goals . . . is imprudent and (we believe) inappropriate public policy for a society deeply divided about the morality of abortion.
>
> Apart from the implications of our society's divisive abortion debate, we have serious reservations about the use of abortion as a means of achieving public health goals of prevention. Preventing the birth of someone who would have an illness or disability is morally different from preventing illness or disability in persons already living. (p. 2418)

Although the AMA panel may have been correct in regard to compelled action to prevent the birth of a child with HIV infection, it is certainly arguable that women who know themselves to be infected and their partners have a duty to exercise special care to avoid conception and birth of a child whose life will be both short and dominated by health concerns (see Howe, 1990, for a sensitive discussion of questions of reproductive choice when a parent is infected with HIV). Regardless of the proper ethical calculus, though, women with HIV infection tend to behave as if such a duty does not exist. The decision of HIV-positive women whether to terminate pregnancy is related more highly to pregnancy-related variables (e.g., history of abortion, planning for a pregnancy) than perception of risk of vertical transmission (Selwyn et al., 1989).

Pregnant women with HIV infection do have somewhat diminished autonomy in the law, with possible deleterious effects on their own health as well as on that of their unborn child. Development of treatment for HIV-infected pregnant women and prevention or treatment of HIV infection in their fetuses has been impeded by a federal rule requiring paternal as well as maternal consent for admission into research in which fetuses are at least incidentally involved (DHHS, 1991b, §46.207[b]). Specifically, the regulations on research on fetuses have delayed and then interfered with clinical trials for AZT treatment of HIV-infected pregnant women and their fetuses (see Kolata, 1991). It is ironic that pregnant women have less autonomy in decision making about fetal research than about child research (for which permission of only one parent is necessary), even though their own health may be impaired by a lack of access to clinical trials.

Because of the preference of some to avoid the birth of a child who may have HIV infection and because of the desire to facilitate early treatment, the Institute of Medicine (IoM, 1991) favors *voluntary* screening of pregnant women in high-prevalence areas. The IoM does not favor newborn screening, in part because treatment of newborns is of unknown toxicity, especially for those infants who in fact are not infected.

The AMA (1990) panel took a more expansive position. It advocated voluntary screening of not only pregnant women but also newborns. This policy was argued to be consistent with the following goals:

(1) to advance the national campaign to educate the public about HIV disease and how it can be prevented; (2) to enhance the current and future reproductive choices of women; (3) to identify women and newborns who can benefit from medical advances in the clinical management of HIV infection; and (4) to allow proper obstetrical treatment of women infected with HIV. (AMA, 1990, p. 2417)

The AMA panel suggested that the usual dominant values in medical ethics of respect for personal choice and protection of confidentiality are especially important in crafting policy in regard to pregnancy and AIDS. The panel noted the number and depth of the various privacy interests at stake, including reproductive choice and avoidance of "social risk" (AMA, 1990, p. 2418). Even with that assessment, though, the AMA panel hedged in its calculation of the projected costs and benefits of its recommendations by noting that the guidelines may change if the technology of intrapartum intervention is altered significantly. Such a qualification is endemic to public health and law, in which the tradition is to rely heavily on expert evidence (Melton, 1988b).

Who Must Know?

The Problem of Confidentiality

A variant of the question of the limits of autonomy in matters relating to HIV infection is the problem of the limits of confidentiality. Although informed consent typically is analyzed apart from confidentiality, both problems involve questions of maintenance of control over one's person (in regard to confidentiality, control over personal information). Nonetheless, the issues are separable to the degree that, as already noted, authority to consent to diagnosis and treatment does not necessarily imply control over access to information obtained in the process of obtaining such services. By the same token, the patient ordinarily retains some expectations of privacy even when a third party (e.g., a parent) has authorized the health services that the patient has received.

Nonetheless, it is clear that minors generally lack the level of privacy that is available to adults, even if children and youths also find privacy important (see Melton, 1983). Not only do parents have control over a child's medical and educational records in most circumstances, but children also often are subject to infringement of the privacy of their associations and personal effects by parents and by the state acting through school officials.

Apart from the question about whether independent privacy interests of minors are to be recognized, the issue arises about who else has a legitimate need to know a child's HIV status. Accordingly, both parents and child may find themselves unable to control release of information about serostatus to school and health officials.[5] Moreover, even if an adolescent's confidentiality against his or her parents is recognized in general, HIV seropositivity may be sufficiently serious that it warrants release to them so that they can respond adequately to their child's medical and psychological needs.

Parents

A common question in treatment and research related to AIDS concerns the degree to which minors can preserve confidentiality against their parents. The answer is clearest when the service relates to treatment or prevention of substance abuse. Federal substance-abuse regulations require all programs receiving federal funds to refrain from disclosing information that would identify the client as a substance user (for a comprehensive, practically oriented review of the federal regulations, see Brooks, 1990). Under those regulations, the young client must always sign any form for release of information about him or her, even if the release is to the parents.[6]

Under other circumstances, the question of adolescent confidentiality turns at least in part on the identity of the party who has power to consent to treatment. If parents are in such a position, they ordinarily should have access to their child's medical records so that they can make informed judgments about treatment, unless they explicitly waive such a right.[7] On the other hand, if the adolescent is the party giving consent, then the inquiry must continue to the question of the purpose of recognition of authority to consent. If the purpose is to respect liberty and privacy, then the youth should have control over information arising from the health services. If it is simply to facilitate treatment (even in the context of perceived resistance to services by parents), then, as already noted, parents may need to know information about their child's seropositivity in order to provide adequate care, and clinicians may have a duty to inform parents about the services that are being rendered and the reason for them.

School Personnel

Although the question of parents' access to information about their adolescent child's serostatus may be the most difficult (especially in circumstances where their interests often are adverse; e.g., runaways and "throwaways"), issues about release of such information to third parties outside the family have attracted more controversy. For example, there has been a debate about whether school officials have a need to know pupils' HIV serostatus. South Carolina (1988/1990) has taken the most intrusive stance in this regard; it requires health professionals to release such information to the school.

The American Academy of Pediatrics (AAP) and CDC have taken the position that the release of information to the school should be decided on a case-by-case basis, but that in any event, knowledge of a child's HIV status should be restricted to "the minimum [number] needed to assure proper care of the child and to detect situations in which the potential for transmission may increase" (AAP, 1986,

p. 431; see also AAP, 1987). Such a policy may be more intrusive than necessary. As a leading authority on the issue as it pertains to college health has argued:

> The concept of a "need to know" among institutional officers is relevant only when someone's need for services demands that the provider be aware of the situation. To say in more general terms that certain officers must know the identity of students with HIV infection on the campus, for example, is more often to justify purposeless talk than to provide useful intervention. *It is difficult to show any cogent reason for most administrators to have any specific knowledge of students or colleagues with HIV infection.* (Keeling, 1988, p. 19, emphasis in original)

Although some have contended that knowledge about a child's serostatus is educationally useful, there is no obvious reason why such knowledge should affect an individual educational plan. The only educational benefit might be greater empathy by teachers, especially if the child appears to be on a path of otherwise unexplained regression.

Child Care Workers, Foster Parents, and Adoptive Parents

Similar issues have arisen in regard to children's caretakers, whether foster or adoptive parents or child care workers. CDC (1985c) has recommended that states do routine screening of foster and adoptive children and should inform actual and prospective foster and adoptive parents about the results, because "these parents must make decisions regarding the medical care of the child and must consider the possible social and psychological effects on their families" (p. 520). In this regard, the CDC guidelines appear to go beyond a need to know in order to take proper safety precautions, in that disclosure would not be limited to young children, whose care needs may bring caretakers into contact with the child's bodily fluids (see AAP, 1987).

In contrast, arguing that restrictions on access to programs should not apply "except when their health provider recommends such restrictions to protect them from exposure to infection" (Oliva et al., 1988, p. 588), the Adolescent AIDS Task Force of the San Francisco Department of Public Health concluded:

Confidentiality should be carefully maintained. HIV status should not be disclosed to social service, legal, or probation personnel unless, as determined in the medical review, such disclosure is necessary for the protection of the adolescent or others with whom he or she may have contact. Disclosure to anyone other than the health care provider should occur only with the written consent of the adolescent or on court order when deemed medically necessary. (Oliva, 1988, p. 588)

Given the lack of evidence for transmission of HIV to family members by means other than sexual contact and needle sharing, disclosure of a child's HIV status cannot be justified on the basis of safety alone, especially when a child is able to perform basic hygiene independently. The argument that "social and psychological effects on their families" (CDC, 1985c, p. 520) cannot be considered by prospective foster and adoptive parents without such knowledge, however, may still apply. If a state elects not to provide such information because of the stigma and related exclusion from normal living situations that may arise for wards with HIV infection, fairness dictates that prospective foster and adoptive parents be told that HIV serostatus is a kind of information that will not be disclosed to them. Thus prospective foster and adoptive parents can make a decision about whether they are willing to care for a child who may have HIV infection.

An interesting twist on the issue is provided by the approach that Michigan (1991) has taken. That state's statute providing for protection of confidentiality related to AIDS originally barred disclosure to foster parents of children's HIV-antibody status unless the biological parents agreed or a court order was obtained. The statute was in direct conflict with the state's Child-Placing Agency Licensing Rule, which requires full disclosure to foster parents of their foster child's health history. The conflict was resolved by an amendment to the AIDS law (Michigan, 1991, §333.5131[g]).

Child-Protection Authorities

An additional breach of confidentiality that may occur in the child welfare system is raised in cases of suspected sexual abuse. If a child is found to be HIV positive but there is no evidence of pre- or perinatal transmission, the most plausible explanation is transmission via sexual abuse. Accordingly, to leave no doubt about the legislature's intent in the face of an apparent conflict between the HIV confidentiality statute and the child-abuse reporting law, several states have adopted statutes expressly permitting disclosure of HIV test results for the purpose of reporting suspected child abuse (e.g., Delaware, 1990; Michigan, 1991, § 333.5131[f]; Nevada, 1989; South Carolina, 1988/1990). North Carolina (1990) has gone still further to permit HIV testing without parental consent if the parent refuses such a test and there is reasonable suspicion that the child has an HIV infection or that he or she has been subjected to sexual abuse.

Health Care Workers

One of the greatest controversies over the need to know has pertained to the question of whether health care workers have a right to knowledge about the HIV serostatus of their patients. (Of course, the converse also has been at issue.) At a practical level, the problem of conflict between patients' privacy interests and their need for health care (on the one hand) and health care workers' interest in personal safety (on the other) has been a major stimulus for policy development related to AIDS. Hospital AIDS policies generally have arisen as a result of staff fear, especially in hospitals without experience in caring for patients in concert with AIDS staff protection (Lewis & Montgomery, 1990).[8]

Although the potential conflict of interest between patient and clinician is not specially applicable to children and youth, its context may be, because knowledge of a patient's HIV seropositivity may result in a diminution of access to health care:

> High-risk and HIV-infected youth and adolescent AIDS patients may experience extreme difficulty in obtaining the specialized services they need. Medical care for AIDS patients is costly, and adolescents, particularly if they are not living with their families, often encounter substantial difficulties in obtaining public or private insurance coverage or in locating other sources of free care. Mental health services for the adolescent population are already extremely limited, and few specialized services appropriate to the adolescent population suffering from, or at high risk for, AIDS have been developed. If the existing limitations on adolescents' access to health care generally are exacerbated by HIV-infected status, high-risk adolescents may find it extraordinarily difficult to obtain the medical care and mental health services they need. (English, 1987, p. 6)

Sexual and Drug-Sharing Partners

Perhaps the most controversial issue in ethics and law on AIDS is the question of when, if ever, sexual and drug-sharing partners of HIV-positive individuals should be warned about their partner's serostatus without the consent of the patient (see, e.g., Knapp & VandeCreek, 1990; Totten, Lamb, & Reeder, 1990). This issue has two aspects as applied to the topics of this book. First, prevention of pediatric AIDS is largely a problem of prevention of AIDS among women. Therefore, the question arises about whether there is a special duty to warn women when their sexual partners are infected with HIV (see Howe, 1990, for a discussion). Second, the problem of protection of partners of HIV-positive adolescents is essentially a subset of the broader problem of application of the duty to protect partners of HIV-positive individuals. It differs only in that it is reasonable to believe that, without a specific warning, partners of adolescents are especially unlikely to perceive themselves to be at risk.

As one of us has discussed elsewhere (Melton, 1988b), the applicability of a duty to protect third parties (see *Tarasoff v. Regents of University of California*, 1976) to patients with HIV infection is not clear, and the question has not yet been litigated at an appellate level. Professional opinion seems to be that, if such a duty is applicable, it is narrow; a breach of confidentiality should occur only when other means of eliminating risky behavior by a client with HIV infection have failed or appear likely to fail, and when the partner is unlikely to realize that he or she is at risk (see APA, 1991).

The utility of breaches of confidentiality is likely to be greater in communities with a relatively low prevalence of AIDS. Data from contact tracing in rural South Carolina are illustrative. Public health authorities informed 64 local sexual contacts of HIV-positive men, most of whom had not been previously tested for HIV antibodies, of their partner's seropositive status (Wykoff et al., 1988). Eight of the informed parties were found to be HIV positive. Individuals who were interviewed on 6-month follow-up reported that they had reduced the number of their sexual partners and had increased their use of condoms; these results were obtained among both HIV-positive and HIV-negative individuals.

In another evaluation of contact tracing by the same group in South Carolina (Jones et al., 1990), 132 of 202 people notified were locatable for follow-up. Only 9% thought prior to notification that they had been exposed to HIV, and 87% said that the health department did the right thing in notification.

Should Children With HIV Be the First or Last in Line?

Who Will Pay?

Although the greatest attention has been placed on the limits of confidentiality in cases of HIV infection, the greatest practical policy problem may be availability of geographically and financially accessible services. As applied to adolescents, this problem interacts with the question of consent. Because few adolescents themselves have direct resources for payment of fees for health services, statutes providing for independent consent may do little to increase the availability of services for adolescents desiring them.

For example, Nebraska (1988), like most states, has a law permitting minors to consent independently and confidentially to diagnosis and treatment for sexually transmitted diseases. The very same statute, though, that makes such services confidential also provides that parents are financially liable for them. Apparently, parents are to pay a bill for unknown services for an unknown individual!

Of course, the question of who pays is not limited to minors seeking services on their own. Given the high cost of the approved treatments for AIDS and HIV infection, the problem is a more generic one. It is especially acute for minors who are dependent on the state for payment. Because of this, Congress has approved a special Medicaid waiver for state wards who are HIV infected (Medicare Catastrophic Coverage Act of 1988). People with AIDS, including children, also are eligible for economic support and medical care through Supplemental Security Income.

Access to Conventional Treatment

Even if financing of services is available, services may not be available if discrimination in the distribution of services occurs. In that regard, a network of antidiscrimination statutes may provide some protection against such denial of services. The Supreme Court has held that Section 504 of the Rehabilitation Act of 1973, the law protecting the civil rights of people with disabilities in public-sector contexts, is applicable to infectious diseases (*School Board of Nassau County v. Arline*, 1987). An important, recently enacted law (the Americans With Disabilities Act [ADA] of 1990) applies the same protections in private interstate commerce. The ADA incorporates Rehabilitation Act concepts as applied to individuals with "a physical or mental impairment that substantially limits one or more of the major life activities," who have "a record of such impairment," or who are "regarded as having such an impairment" (ADA, 1990, 3[2]; see Parry, 1991, for citations to Rehabilitation Act cases that probably provide authority for resolution of complaints under ADA).

One particular problem of access to services that is germane to prevention of pediatric AIDS is the availability of services for drug-abusing women, especially those who are pregnant. Many women avoid treatment because of fear of prosecution and loss of child custody. A problem that may be even greater is that the number of slots available for treatment is grossly inadequate, and that many drug treatment programs will not accept pregnant women (General Accounting Office, 1991).

Access to Experimental Treatment

For people who are infected with HIV, a disease for which there is still no cure, hope for a longer life is largely a matter, both individually and collectively, of experimental treatments. Because of reluctance to use children in clinical research, development of treatment for infected or ill children has lagged several years behind that for adults (Nolan, 1990; Valleroy, 1990). Indeed, children were not included at all in studies conducted at AIDS Clinical Trials Units until 1987; adolescents were not included in trials until still later (Hein, 1991). Most of the small number of adolescents who are now enrolled in clinical trials are white males with hemophilia.[9]

The problem of access to clinical trials is not an easy one. On the one hand, clinical trials are the major source of hope for children with HIV infection. Moreover, the results of adult trials cannot be generalized to children, because not only biochemistry but the disease process itself may differ developmentally. For example, *Pneumocystis carinii* pneumonia is a primary infection in children but a reactivation disease in adults (Van Dyke, 1991).

Given the bleak prognosis without access to experimental treatments, it seems implausible that a rational individual would reject the opportunity, even in the face of possible toxic side effects. Accordingly, there may be special reason to trust substituted judgment in the case of children with HIV infection.

On the other hand, however, clinical trials may do more harm than good at times, and children, unlike most adults with HIV infection, are not in a position to provide informed consent.[10] Therefore, it is argued that adults should be first to subject themselves to the risk of exposure to a substance of undemonstrated efficacy, especially when the possibility that it is toxic has not been ruled out. (Of course, a necessary corollary to this approach is that adults also are the first to enjoy benefits of new drugs—a result that conflicts with ethical norms in other contexts, in which children typically are regarded as the first-priority recipients of public aid.)

There are several specific reasons for special care in enrollment of children in clinical trials. First, Phase I drug trials are primarily to detect toxicity, not to demonstrate efficacy, and it seems unfair to place participants who are unable to give informed consent into a situation in which they effectively are the scouts sent to locate danger. Because, though, Phase I results of adults cannot be generalized to children, failure to include children in initial Phase I trials necessarily delays their access to the new treatment if it ultimately is found to be effective.

Second, placebo controls cannot be assumed to be benign in children:[11]

> The monthly placement and several-hour maintenance of an intravenous line in immunocompromised children certainly involves more than minimal risk, and arguably more than a minor increment above minimal risk. Because this level of risk is not directly related to attempts to provide therapy, its justification lies in a delicate balancing of the importance of answering the research question versus the importance of protecting the individual patient-subjects. (Nolan, 1990, pp. 472-473)

Third, medical technology remains at a point where results of trials involving children may subject healthy fetuses and children to treatment with substantial negative side effects. Because the HIV-antibody test is not a reliable indicator of infection in fetuses and infants, overinclusion is a likely problem in clinical trials of HIV treatments for young children.

Fourth, so many children with HIV infection have parents who are either absent or too undependable to follow through on an experimental treatment regimen for their children. Therefore, questions arise about (a) the unjust exclusion of children from access to experimental treatments because of the condition of their parents and the related federal regulations, and (b) the unjust inclusion in risky research of children whose data will be too unreliable to be useful.

To guard against use of foster children as a "convenience sample" for research, federal regulations (DHHS, 1991a) require that permission for state wards' participation in research be granted by not only the legal guardian but also a fourth party not involved in the research project. Although the regulations give no guidance about the selection of such an advocate for the child's interests,[12] they have the potential to be an effective means of protecting children from harm (if the requirement for an advocate is taken seriously).

Nonetheless, state-agency policy is often even more restrictive than the federal regulations. A survey (Martin & Sacks, 1990) of all state child-welfare agencies showed that about 800 children in foster care at one point in time in 1989 were known to be HIV infected. Only 15 were reported to be enrolled in clinical trials. A parallel survey of physicians directing federally funded clinical trials with HIV-infected children identified 69 foster children who had been so enrolled. The pediatric researchers knew of about 200 children who were otherwise eligible for enrollment in their studies but who had been denied admission because permission was not obtainable.

In short, the practice seems to be that foster children are even more likely than children in their homes of origin to be excluded from clinical trials. In view of the availability of procedures for special scrutiny of requests for foster children's participation in research, one must wonder whether the low frequency of involvement of state wards with HIV infection in clinical trials is not an instance of negligence in promoting their health (because of the extra effort required to enroll a foster child in a clinical trial) more than one of diligence in protecting them from harm.

Access to Education

The most visible and highly debated question in regard to infected children's access to services has been outside the health care system. The director of a Harvard project that collects and analyzes legal cases related to AIDS (Gostin, 1990b) has aptly summarized the controversy over admission of children infected with HIV into public schools:

> From the earliest times of the HIV epidemic, exclusion of school children infected with HIV from their classrooms was an issue debated with great emotion. Parents of children infected with HIV sued school boards for denying children state education, giving homebound instruction, or making the child wait for inordinate periods while the board developed a policy. In other cases, HIV-infected children were permitted to attend school, but they were clearly singled out as different by being placed alone in a separate "modular" classroom, by being required to use a separate bathroom and to be accompanied by an adult on all field trips, or even by being isolated inside a glass booth. (p. 2087)

The American Academy of Pediatrics (1986) has concluded that children with HIV infection generally should be permitted to attend school, although the AAP did note that "students who lack control of their body secretions, who display behavior such as biting, or who have open skin sores that cannot be covered require a more restricted school environment until more is known about the transmission of the virus under these conditions" (p. 431; see also CDC, 1985c). The AAP also noted that school attendance may be too risky for some children with HIV infection, because of their susceptibility to infections.

A task force of the American Psychological Association (APA, 1987) has indicated its general support for the AAP and CDC guidelines, although the APA task force also expressed qualms that those guidelines may permit more departures from mainstreaming and breaches of confidentiality than are necessary, given "the nearly non-existent risk of transmission" (p. 4).[13] The task force later specifically recommended revision of the guidelines to give recognition to the lack of evidence for transmission of HIV through saliva. It concluded that "the nearly non-existent risk of infection to classmates does not outweigh the infected child's right to a free and appropriate education in the least restrictive environment" (Task Force on Pediatric AIDS, 1989, p. 260).

Courts have been nearly unanimous in rejecting attempts to exclude children with AIDS from school (e.g., *Board of Education v. Cooperman*, 1987; *District 27 Community School Board v. Board of Education*, 1986; *Doe v. Belleville Public School District*, 1987; *Martinez v. School Board*, 1987; *Ray v. School District*, 1987; *Robertson v. Granite City Community Unit School District No. 9*, 1988; *Thomas v. Atascadero Unified School District*, 1987). Courts' decisions in regard to children with HIV infection follow the precedents established in regard to children with hepatitis-B infection (e.g., *New York State Association for Retarded Children v. Carey*, 1979).

Indeed, courts typically not only have rendered decisions supportive of children with HIV infection in regular schools, but have used strong language in doing so. The words of one federal district judge are illustrative:

> It is difficult for the Court to imagine anything more traumatic for a child than going to school and being placed in a classroom by himself, not being allowed to play with other children, and not even [being] allowed to eat with his classmates. (*Robertson v. Granite City Community Unit School District No. 9*, 1988, p. 1005)

The legal foundation for injunctions against removal of children with HIV infection from regular schools has been diverse. Perhaps the most obvious rationale is that the Education for All Handicapped Children Act of 1974 (EAHCA) mandates that children with disabilities receive a free, appropriate education in the least restrictive environment. The EAHCA, however, has been held to apply to children with AIDS only if their educational performance is impaired by the HIV infection itself (*Doe v. Belleville Public School District*, 1987; *Robertson v. Granite City Community Unit School District No. 9*, 1988). (Note that, as in *Robertson*, the pupil may be covered by the EAHCA because of other conditions, but an exclusion from school because of the HIV infection would not be barred by the EAHCA in such a case.) Even if children with AIDS are not covered by the EAHCA, though, their exclusion from school still will be prohibited in most circumstances by the Rehabilitation Act (as also held in *Doe* and *Robertson*) and the Americans With Disabilities Act. The broader statutes actually present a more favorable context for plaintiffs, because they need not exhaust administrative remedies before appealing to a court for an injunction against removal of a child from school.

Right to a Family Environment

Although the attempts to remove children with HIV infection from school have been tragic, an even more basic issue is presented by the right of children with HIV infection (like all children) to a family environment (UN Convention on the Rights of the Child, 1989, preamble and art. 20). It has been estimated that New York City alone will need to find homes for 40,000 children orphaned by AIDS in the 1990s (Heagarty, 1991). More than 20% of hospitalizations of children with AIDS at Harlem Hospital are the product of social problems rather than medical needs (Hegarty et al., 1988; see also Kemper & Forsyth, 1988). The cost is extreme; hospital care in such cases averaged 339 days, compared with 89 days for children living at home.

In the face of such demand, the cost of hospital-based boarding arrangements, and community prejudice, some policymakers have even called for a return to orphanages as options in child welfare. Others have not gone so far, but they have advocated unconventional foster care arrangements that differ substantially from a normal family environment. For example, Boston City Hospital ("Boston City Hospital," 1986) established a home for children with AIDS and some of their mothers. The hospital originally planned to develop the residence away from the hospital, but the in-hospital location was chosen in order to avoid neighborhood opposition. Although the result was certainly less restrictive and expensive than a regular inpatient ward, one may reasonably question whether a "home" in a hospital is really respectful of the dignity of its residents.

Still, one must recognize that the challenge to child-welfare authorities is extraordinary. At the same time that emergency conditions exist in the child-protection system as a whole (see U.S. Advisory Board, 1990), overburdened caseworkers must find and support foster families willing to undertake the care of children with HIV infection. Even if potential foster parents are not themselves deterred by irrational beliefs about the risk of contracting AIDS from a child for whom they are caring, they may have realistic concerns about the psychological costs of dealing with community reaction and the special needs for care of a child with HIV infection. (To the extent that either such needs are unlikely to appear quickly or the family feels comfortable in meeting them, the significance of confidentiality becomes especially profound.) If an adequate number of foster families is to be available, child-welfare agencies will have to arrange for subsidies to compensate foster parents for the special demands that are placed upon them. Agencies also will have to provide foster parents with other forms of support, including respite care and training, if state wards with HIV infection are to be assured of a living situation that approximates a family environment.

Should AIDS Educators Be Preachers?

Morality and AIDS Prevention

As policymakers struggle not only to make adequate care and treatment available for people with AIDS but also to prevent HIV infection altogether, a persistent tension has been present between (a) the desire to promote public health and support a humane, dignified life for people with HIV infection and (b) the desire to avoid symbolic approval of the behavior that led to the infection. At least in regard to IV drug use, such a conflict occurs even when public health authorities do not fall into the morally bankrupt position of assignment of responsibility for their illness to people with HIV infection. Although the AIDS epidemic may have resulted in a new legitimation of conservative social norms "for monogamy, constancy and predictability" (Price, 1989, p. 14), no one deserves AIDS!

No more difficult conflict between facilitating safer behavior and symbolic approval of illegal, risky behavior has been present than in the debate about whether to support needle exchange programs. The empirical evidence thus far suggests that the conflict is hypothetical: Encouragement of safer drug-taking behavior appears not to stimulate new drug use, but it does offer a step toward entrance into treatment and risk reduction (Des Jarlais & Friedman, 1988). Nonetheless, symbolic effects are difficult to document, and that such effects do occur is accordingly difficult to refute persuasively without a substantial history of evaluation of the operation of needle exchange projects—a history that currently does not exist.

AIDS Education in Three States

Although concern about needle exchange programs is understandable, analogous debate about other aspects of AIDS prevention seems to reflect a willingness to threaten the lives of people in order to protect moral norms that are far from universally held. The policy responses that have occurred can be illustrated by comparing three states' legislative approaches to AIDS education.

Most straightforwardly, Iowa (1988/1989a) requires development and dissemination of a "medically correct" AIDS education program for public schools. The Iowa statute also mandates AIDS education for all primary and secondary school pupils whose parents consent to such a program.

In contrast, the Texas legislature (Human Immunodeficiency Virus Services Act of 1989) has made clear that it views AIDS education as less a straightforward exercise in public health than an opportunity to reinforce traditional morality:

> All materials in the education programs intended for persons under 18 years of age shall emphasize sexual abstinence before marriage and fidelity in marriage as the expected standard in terms of public health and the most effective ways to prevent HIV infection, sexually transmitted diseases, and unwanted pregnancies and shall state that homosexual conduct is not an acceptable lifestyle and is a criminal offense under Section 21.06 of the Penal Code. (art. 4419b-4, § 1.03[j])[14]

Missouri (1988/1991) has taken a middle approach that is more cautious than necessary but not quite as restrictive as the Texas program. The Missouri legislature directed the state health department to develop a "medically correct" and "age specific" curriculum to be used at the discretion of individual public schools. The curriculum is to be limited, however, to secondary school students. In authorizing the program, Missouri legislators also required the program planners to "stress moral responsibility in and restraint from sexual activity and avoidance of controlled substance abuse."

The Promotion of Ignorance
in the Name of Morality

Perhaps the most objectionable response to AIDS prevention has been the resistance, purportedly grounded in traditional morality, to not only diffusion but gathering of information that may be helpful in reducing the incidence of AIDS. Conservatives led by Senator Helms of North Carolina and Congressman Dannemeyer of California have been successful in suppressing surveys of teenagers about their sexual behavior (including research that had already been approved for funding by peer review panels) and in withholding millions of brochures on AIDS and its prevention (Barnes, 1991; Wilcox, 1990). Such unprecedented promotion of ignorance—particularly when ignorance can have lethal consequences—is impossible to justify.

Recognizing the political obstacles to development of the basic knowledge needed for an effective AIDS prevention program, a panel of the National Academy of Sciences has recommended exemption of AIDS research from the Paperwork Reduction Act, which has provided the legal authority for the Office of Management and the Budget to slow down the effort to increase knowledge relevant to prevention of AIDS (Turner, Miller, & Moses, 1989). Although this step would remove one obstacle, considerable persistence in the political arena will be necessary if even the rudiments of AIDS prevention strategies aimed at adolescents are to be carried out.

Is Fear a Legitimate Basis for Public Policy?

Unfortunately, the debate on AIDS often has been guided more by irrational fear than realistic concerns. AIDS is not logical; it is hard to believe that a contagious disease so deadly is transmitted by such limited means. The result has been not only that children have been targeted removal for school without any real rationale but also that resources sometimes have been diverted toward mass screening programs of low-prevalence populations (e.g., testing of applicants for marriage licenses, testing of health care workers) at the same time that more cost-effective prevention programs are underfunded. AIDS policy too often is based on unwise decisions that are the product of fear of casual contagion.

Ruling on the constitutionality of a public mental retardation agency's plan for HIV testing of its staff, a federal district court in Nebraska was caustic in its assessment of the justification for the policy:

The evidence leads to the conclusion that the policy was prompted by concerns about the AIDS virus, formulated with little or erroneous medical knowledge, and is a constitutionally impermissible reaction to a devastating disease with no known cure. The risk of transmission of the disease from the staff to the clients at the agency is minuscule, trivial, extremely low, extraordinarily low, theoretical, and approaches zero. Such a risk does not justify the implementation of such a sweeping policy that ignores and violates the staff members' constitutional rights. (*Glover v. Eastern Nebraska Community Office of Retardation,* 1988, p. 250)

Even if the actual risk is "minuscule, trivial, extremely low, extraordinarily low, theoretical, and approach[ing] zero," the question remains whether the more important factor is perceived risk. For example, even if the mass screening of health care workers cannot be justified in terms of its cost-effectiveness in preventing HIV infection, a plausible argument can be made that such a policy is necessary because of the loss of public confidence in the health care system that may result if patients believe, even if erroneously, that they are at significant risk of contracting an HIV infection from their physician or dentist. Similarly, a pragmatist may wonder whether the cost to children's education of mass boycotts, as occurred in some communities early in the AIDS epidemic, can be justified by the protection of the rights of one child with AIDS.

Our own view is that, despite the short-term avoidance of social conflict and accompanying loss of productivity in the various systems of public service, health professionals, school officials, and other community leaders have a duty not to buckle under community pressure emanating from a lack of information, erroneous calculations of risk, or simple prejudice. Our conclusion is based on two premises, one that is purely pragmatic and another that is basic to public morality and constitutional rights.

First, apart from the personal suffering of the individuals who lose access to public services as a result of fear-based policies, there is substantial long-term social cost of failure to address the actual realities of AIDS and HIV infection. That school boycotts no longer occur is a testament at least in part to the courts and school officials who refused to use public opinion as a rationale to deprive individual children of an education and to stigmatize them further when no objective rationale existed for such discriminatory action. As indi-

cated by the naming of major federal AIDS legislation after Ryan White
(Ryan White Comprehensive AIDS Resources Emergency Act of 1990),
the apparent dampening of public hysteria is also the product of
courageous action by some children with AIDS and their families
who were willing to place themselves in the center of public attention in order to protect their own rights and those of other children
and families faced not only with a life-threatening illness but also
with mean-spirited responses of some public officials and members
of the general public.

Failure by public officials to take affirmative action to reduce prejudice may sustain it. For example, a phone survey of 16- to 19-year-
olds in Massachusetts in 1986 (Strunin et al., 1988) found that nearly
one fourth of the respondents favored exclusion from school of children with AIDS. The proportion was much higher among those youth
who had incorrect beliefs about the means of contracting the disease.
Nearly two fifths of those who believed that HIV could be transmitted
through contract with eating utensils (a belief held by 42% of the
sample who expressed an opinion) supported exclusion of infected
children. Exclusion also was favored by 45% of those who believed
that HIV could be transmitted through the air (a belief held by about
one fifth of the sample) and 62% of the small group who thought
that HIV could be communicated by shaking hands (4% of the sample).
It is easy to see how acting as if fictions were true could sustain such
beliefs and result in increasingly irrational and discriminatory policy.

The courts' role in fostering long-term community harmony and
diminishing community fear through action that may be unpopular
in the short term is illustrated by the statement of a federal district
court in Illinois:

> Given the volatility of the issue, it would seem that returning Jason to
> a normal classroom setting would demonstrate to the public that this
> problem must be dealt with in a rational fashion, and our collective
> knowledge, based on a reasonable medical certainty, indicates that a
> child in Jason's condition poses no significant threat to his classmates.
> Furthermore, it is clear that this controversy has evoked unrest in the
> Granite City Community and placing Jason back in a regular class-
> room will, at least temporarily, end this controversy. Hopefully, in the
> time between issuance of this injunction and a trial on the merits, the
> District and the Board can continue with their previous efforts at
> educating the public and allaying any unfounded or misguided fears

they may have. Therefore, the Court finds that the public interest will
not be harmed by issuance of an injunction. (*Robertson v. Granite City
Community Unit School District No. 9*, 1988, p. 1006)

The direct significance of such judicial action was demonstrated
in a survey of administrators of Southern California school districts
(Liss, 1989). Although the sample size was too small for statistical
analysis, administrators appeared to show less concern for community reaction and legal liability, more concern about the needs of
children with HIV infections, and more openness about the topic
after the first case in California in which a court upheld the right of
infected children to attend school (*Phipps v. Saddleback Valley Unified
School District*, 1986).

Second, even if the long-term social calculus of discriminatory policies was positive, public officials still should reject such policies
because they are wrong. The fact that an individual has a disease
should not be cause in itself to treat him or her as a leper. (The irony
of the analogy is intentional.) A debilitating, life-threatening illness
creates its own kind of prison, but that fact does not diminish person-
hood. A weak body diminishes dignity only if society permits it to
do so, and government should not collude in action that degrades
any of its citizens. As the Supreme Court has noted in other contexts,
"private biases may be outside the reach of the law [in a society that
has made equal protection a fundamental principle in its law], but
the law cannot, directly or indirectly, give them effect" (*Palmore v.
Sidoti*, 1984, p. 433).

The Supreme Court has recognized further that public policy has
turned, in general, toward broad legislation to prevent and remedi-
ate the social and personal costs of discrimination based purely in
fear. Prior to the enactment of the Americans With Disabilities Act
(1990), the Court affirmed that Section 504 of the Rehabilitation Act
of 1973 applied to persons with contagious diseases:

By amending the definition of "handicapped individual" to include
not only those who are actually physically impaired, but also those
who are regarded as impaired and who, as a result, are substantially
limited in a major life activity, Congress acknowledged that society's
accumulated myths and fears about disability and disease are as
handicapping as are the physical limitations that flow from actual
impairment. . . . The Act is carefully structured to replace such reflex-

ive reactions to actual or perceived handicaps with actions based on reasoned and medically sound judgments. . . . The fact that some persons who have contagious diseases may pose a serious health threat to others under certain circumstances does not justify excluding from the coverage of the Act all persons with actual or perceived contagious diseases. Such exclusion would mean that those accused of being contagious would never have the opportunity to have their condition evaluated in light of medical evidence and a determination made as to whether they were "otherwise qualified." Rather, they would be vulnerable to discrimination on the basis of mythology—precisely the type of injury Congress sought to prevent. (*School Board v. Arline*, 1987, pp. 284-285)

The reference to "medical evidence" indicates the particular duty that health professionals have to avoid stimulating or sustaining fear that may provoke prejudice and discrimination and, indeed, to promote reasoned, humane policies. Unfortunately, scientists have not always been so careful. The implication that AIDS had been transmitted through casual contagion was left in the *Journal of the American Medical Association* in an early report of pediatric cases of AIDS (Oleske et al., 1983). Such an implication, which was simply sloppy science, may still underlie the fears of many in the general public (see Batchelor, 1988).

Ultimately, eradication of the stigma attached to HIV infection may be necessary for effective prevention (see Herek & Glunt, 1988). The duty to lead toward such social change may be much more important than other ethical matters (e.g., questions about application of *Tarasoff*) that have been in the forefront of discussion of ethical and legal issues related to AIDS. Both as individuals and as organizations, health professionals can do much to ensure that the stigma of pediatric and adolescent AIDS is not itself disabling.

Notes

1. Directly germane to the question whether parents can be depended upon to guard the interests of children with AIDS is evidence of noncompliance with the treatment regimen by a substantial proportion of parents whose ill children were enrolled in a clinical trial (McKinney et al., 1991). Parents' own illness and substance abuse may interfere with their ability to assist in their children's health care.

PEDIATRIC AND ADOLESCENT AIDS

2. That many such qualifiers have to be added suggests that the question of parent-child relations in cases of AIDS is not so simple. Clearly, the assumption that all such characteristics are generally present in a particular case often will be erroneous even if perhaps widely held.

3. Levin et al. (1991) also found that health care professionals overestimate the prevalence of HIV infection among children of women with AIDS.

4. Comparable questions arise in regard to the problem of whether women who are HIV infected should be encouraged or compelled to use contraception in order not to transmit the virus. The AMA (1990) panel discussed below reached a negative conclusion on this question, as it did on advocacy of abortion.

5. The discussion herein certainly does not exhaust the circumstances in which either the privacy of people with AIDS may be threatened or the law may offer special protection to them. Rather, our discussion focuses on the problems of confidentiality that are in some way specific to pediatric or adolescent HIV infection. Compare Gray and Melton (1985); see also Melton (1990), discussing certificates of confidentiality for research data.

6. Under the regulations, whether a minor can consent independently to diagnosis and treatment of substance abuse is a matter of state law.

7. The validity of such a waiver may still be in question. Can the parents foresee the circumstances that may arise in treatment sufficiently well to make an informed decision to waive their right of access? Probably, though, such a waiver is possible, because parents may make a judgment in the light of the general information available to them that their child's treatment would be more effective if his or her privacy was respected. They also may perceive such boundaries as consistent with their values in child rearing.

8. The answer to the problem of preservation of health care workers' safety without special stigmatization of patients with AIDS is the adoption of universal precautions. Such an approach minimizes the risk of exposure to not only HIV but also other blood-borne pathogens.

9. As Hein (1991) pointed out, studies of adolescent behavior potentially leading to HIV infection and of the epidemiology of HIV infection among adolescents are even less common, at least partly because of a lack of attention by federal research authorities. Most notably and outrageously, Secretary of Health and Human Services Louis Sullivan recently took the unprecedented step of rescinding a grant for a large-scale study of adolescent sexual behavior (see Barnes, 1991).

10. Note that, de facto if not de jure, this argument may not apply to adolescents, who have been particularly excluded from clinical trials.

11. Now that zidovudine has been approved for therapeutic use for both children and adults, there is good reason to question whether placebo controls can ever be justified. Absent a compelling justification to the contrary, the standard treatment rather than no treatment should be the control condition.

12. Possible sources of knowledgeable advocates would be organizations of foster parents and advocacy organizations for children with disabilities and development of health care for children in poverty.

13. A similar position was articulated by the Surgeon General's workshop on children with HIV infection (Department of Health & Human Services, 1987).

14. A still more detailed directive to the Texas Board of Health on the moral content of AIDS education is found in the Human Immunodeficiency Act of 1989, art. 4419b-5, which focuses on "self-control," with "abstinence from sexual intercourse outside of lawful marriage . . . [as] the expected societal standard for school-age unmarried persons."

EIGHT

Research Priorities

Issues Regarding Infected Children and Adolescents

The working group of the Department of Health and Human Services (DHHS) Special Initiative on Pediatric AIDS (Novello et al., 1989) has outlined several major medical research goals, including further empirical examination of epidemiological issues, diagnostic techniques, transmission routes and precise timing of HIV infection, disease progression, and the effectiveness of medical treatment modalities. Other groups have focused predominantly on psychosocial research needs (e.g., Coates et al., 1987; Task Force on Pediatric AIDS, 1989), including AIDS prevention, psychosocial correlates of HIV infection, and, among others, the consideration of cultural and ethnic factors in the conduct of research. The purpose of this section is to highlight specific psychosocial research needs and priorities in four areas: epidemiology, diagnosis and assessment of psychosocial sequelae, the clinical course of HIV infection and AIDS, and psychosocial intervention.

Epidemiological Issues

Recent advances in medicine and science have answered many important questions regarding the epidemiology of HIV infection and AIDS. For instance, HIV transmission routes have been well documented and delineated. Seroprevalence studies also have documented rising rates of HIV infection among IV drug users, heterosexual women, children, and minorities. There are many additional epidemiological issues about the long-term sequelae of HIV infection, however, that can be answered only with time. Unfortunately, many of these unanswered questions pertain specifically to infants, children, and adolescents, whose disease progression is rapid and for whom death is imminent.

Several epidemiological issues are germane to researchers interested in delineating the psychosocial aspects of pediatric AIDS. For instance, what is the prevalence rate of neuropsychological and developmental deficits secondary to HIV infection and AIDS in young children? Which subgroups among older children and adolescents are at significantly elevated risk of acquiring HIV infection, and what is the rate of infection within each transmission mode? In light of its relationship to risky behaviors (e.g., increased sexual activity and IV drug use), what impact will the present crack-cocaine epidemic have on the incidence of AIDS among adolescents? Answers to these questions might help direct the future development of primary, secondary, and tertiary intervention efforts.

Diagnosis and Assessment
of Psychosocial Sequelae

Delineation of the psychosocial concomitants of HIV infection and AIDS in children and adolescents continues to be a much needed area of investigation. For instance, what is the impact of HIV infection on the social, behavioral, and cognitive functioning of infants, children, and adolescents? Are observed social, behavioral, and cognitive sequelae the products of HIV infection or of other secondary factors (e.g., poor prenatal care, prematurity, social isolation, drug use, a caretaker with progressive disease process)?

It also seems imperative that we examine existing diagnostic and assessment tools used with other chronically ill populations to determine their utility and relevance to children with AIDS. Is there a need to develop more valid and reliable methods for detecting psychosocial problems in young children with AIDS, or are existing instruments adequate? In exploring the utility of existing psychological measurements for children with AIDS, we need to work toward developing appropriate norms on such instruments, particularly for children representing ethnic minority groups.

The range of psychological impairment or disability in children with AIDS and its relationship to disease progression also warrant empirical examination. What demographic, individual, or family characteristics contribute to successful psychosocial adaptation to AIDS? Moreover, although vertically infected children have an extremely poor prognosis at present, the discovery of life-prolonging medical treatments will bring into sharp focus the need for research on compliance with medical regimens. Also, although most vertically infected children now die before they enroll in school, life-prolonging interventions will necessitate coordination and evaluation of appropriate psychoeducational programming for this population.

Of course, pediatric AIDS is unusual in that more than one family member may be affected at the same time. For instance, many mothers have to struggle not only with their own diagnosis but also with that of their newborn child. Considering that many mothers of HIV-infected children are IV drug users or interact frequently (and sexually) with those who are, the nature and degree of psychological difficulties may be quite extensive. Many of these individuals are already dealing with traumatic situations; the birth of a child with HIV infection may increase their vulnerability and susceptibility to depression, stress, social isolation, and other psychological difficulties (see Chapter 6). Therefore, it is important to include indices of family adaptation in studies of children with AIDS so that the relationship between family functioning and child adaptation can be examined.

The Clinical Course of HIV and AIDS in Children and Adolescents

From a psychological perspective, there are several areas regarding the clinical course of HIV that warrant exploration. First, researchers might examine the role of various cofactors in the progression of HIV infection and AIDS. For instance, does maternal IV drug use or the presence of other viral infections during pregnancy subsequently lead to a more rapid progression of disease in HIV-infected offspring? Second, the relationship between psychological factors (e.g., stress) and immune functioning in infants, children, and adolescents with HIV infection or AIDS remains unclear (Task Force on Pediatric AIDS, 1989). This seems to be a particularly important research need in light of the hypothesized relationship between heightened and recurrent stress and compromised immune functioning (Kiecolt-Glaser & Glaser, 1987).

Third, as noted in Chapter 1, HIV infection in the central nervous system (CNS) occurs sooner in the disease process and more frequently in children than in adults, perhaps because of the immaturity and plasticity of the child's developing nervous system. A more comprehensive understanding of HIV infection in CNS disease is necessary, however, so that remedial efforts can be undertaken to avert its debilitating effects. For instance, what are the precise timing and cellular targets of HIV infection in the developing brain? What short- and long-term changes in CNS functioning, brain growth, physical development, neurocognitive functioning, and social development occur over time in children with HIV infection and AIDS? Fourth, more information about the clinical course of HIV and AIDS in adolescents is needed. Because adolescents have "fallen between the cracks" with respect to epidemiology and clinical trials, we presently do not know the true extent of the AIDS problem in this subgroup, nor do we know the degree to which factors unique to this age group (e.g., hormonal changes) affect disease progression.

Psychosocial Interventions

Recent research suggests that psychological factors may moderate various aspects of immune functioning. Indeed, in their review of the literature, Kiecolt-Glaser and Glaser (1987) postulated a strong association between immunosuppression and recurrent stressful experiences. Heightened and sustained levels of stress, for instance, have been found to be associated with the expression of symptomatology in individuals with Epstein-Barr virus and herpes. One implication of these research findings for those with HIV infection or AIDS is that effective stress management techniques may slow viral progression or even enhance immune functioning. For example, a nutritionally balanced diet, exercise, life-style modifications, and other social-environmental factors may slow the progression of AIDS symptomatology (Antoni et al., 1990; Coates et al., 1987). Despite this promising line of inquiry, no empirical studies have been conducted to examine the efficacy of psychosocial interventions with children living with AIDS.

Because vertical transmission of HIV has become the predominant precursor to AIDS among children, primary prevention efforts are directed necessarily toward adult behaviors. Secondary and tertiary prevention efforts in children and adolescents, however, must not be neglected. Specifically, educational programs for young children to increase their awareness of risky behaviors might be designed, implemented, and evaluated. Existing educational and behavioral interventions for adolescents and women of childbearing age also might be assessed. Moreover, researchers might evaluate empirically the relative contribution of positive health practices (e.g., diet, exercise, stress management) to disease management and progression.

Several authors have noted that adolescents with HIV infection have had limited access to clinical trials (e.g., Futterman & Hein, 1991; Gayle & D'Angelo, 1991). Limited access has occurred because pediatric research protocols usually include children under 13 years of age, and adult research protocols exclude individuals under 18 years of age. Future research efforts must be geared toward developing and evaluating adolescent health care models. Helping HIV-infected adolescents reduce or eliminate ongoing risky behavior is a priority.

Additional research needs include the evaluation of psychosocial interventions with diverse cultural and ethnic groups, an examination of the relationship between pharmacological interventions and psychosocial problems (e.g., anxiety, depression) in children and adolescents, and the application and evaluation of multisystemic approaches (Henggeler & Borduin, 1990) to treating children with AIDS and their families.

Issues Regarding Noninfected Children and Adolescents

AIDS Knowledge and Attitudes

In light of the generally high levels of knowledge about AIDS among teenagers and young adults, future research should delineate the characteristics of youths who have low levels of knowledge. Such delineation requires evaluation of the moderators (e.g., gender, ethnicity) and mediators (e.g., intelligence, social competence, family relations) of AIDS knowledge and will facilitate the cost-effective application of educational efforts. Similarly, studies of the link between AIDS knowledge and risk-taking behavior should include more complex analyses to assess third-variable explanations for findings. For example, perhaps an association between AIDS knowledge and use of condoms is attributable primarily to their conjoint relationship with intelligence, social competence, or social desirability. In addition, investigations should evaluate AIDS knowledge among groups of youths that largely have been ignored and whose risk-taking behaviors may place them at increased risk of infection (e.g., delinquents, substance abusers, homeless youths).

Multivariate methods also can be used to examine the moderators and mediators of misconceptions about AIDS. Additionally, however, the use of qualitative methods might provide a better understanding of *why* certain youths hold misconceptions. For example, interviewers can ask follow-up questions regarding a youth's expressed belief that HIV can be transmitted through classroom contact.

Youths (in the same manner as adults) hold negative attitudes toward AIDS and persons with AIDS, and such attitudes probably are associated with the deadly nature of the disease and the link between AIDS and groups of persons who already are stigmatized (Herek & Glunt, 1988). Although it seems unreasonable to expect people not to hold a negative attitude toward a deadly disease such as AIDS, methods of attenuating negative attitudes toward AIDS victims should be evaluated for moral (e.g., human compassion) and social policy (e.g., funding initiatives) purposes.

Adolescents' Sexual Behavior

Little is known about the sexual activities of adolescents, aside from the time of first intercourse. In particular, frequency and prevalence data are lacking for specific high-risk sexual behaviors such as anal intercourse among homosexual and heterosexual youths. Surveys of adolescent sexual behaviors should be comprehensive in scope and attend to moderating variables such as gender, ethnicity, and age; such data are a prerequisite to selective targeting of prevention efforts at adolescents who are in greatest need.

In light of the multiple correlates of heterosexual activity and condom use (encompassing biological, cognitive, peer, and family variables), it seems likely that similar social-ecological factors will be linked with high-risk sexual behaviors in teens. Hence, prevention and intervention should not focus on limited aspects of the youth's ecology (e.g., "just say no") but should provide broad-based and comprehensive services to be maximally effective. Most importantly, prevention and intervention services should be specified well and evaluated rigorously, including determinations of client characteristics linked with positive behavior change.

Adolescents' IV Drug Use

Adolescents who use IV drugs present a myriad of serious psychosocial difficulties, one of which is the increased probability of contracting and spreading HIV. In light of these psychosocial difficulties, treatment should aim to eliminate substance use. Unfortunately, no treatments of adolescent substance abuse have proven effective in controlled studies, though several multifaceted approaches are promising. Likewise, other types of antisocial behavior in adolescents have proven quite recalcitrant to treatment. Such findings suggest that effective risk-reduction strategies for adolescent IV drug users will be difficult to develop. Nevertheless, as suggested by uncontrolled outreach efforts reviewed earlier, it may be possible to specify particular treatment components that influence drug-use behavior in this population.

References

Agnew, R. (1985). Social control theory and delinquency: A longitudinal test. *Criminology, 23,* 47-61.

AIDS victim kept from school in Indiana. (1985, August 1). *The New York Times,* p. A15.

Amadori, A., DeRossi, A., Giaquinto, C., Faulkner-Valle, G., Zacchello, F., & Chieco-Bianchi, L. (1988). In-vitro production of HIV-specific antibody in children at risk of AIDS. *Lancet, 1,* 852-854.

American Academy of Pediatrics, Committee on Infectious Diseases. (1987). Health guidelines for the attendance in day-care and foster care settings of children infected with human immunodeficiency virus. *Pediatrics, 79,* 466-469.

American Academy of Pediatrics, Committees on School Health and Infectious Diseases. (1986). School attendance of children and adolescents with human T lymphotropic virus III/lymphadenopathy-associated virus infection. *Pediatrics, 77,* 430-432.

American Medical Association. (1987). *Ethical issues involved in the growing AIDS crisis* (Report of the Council on Ethical and Judicial Affairs). Chicago: Author.

American Medical Association, Working Group on HIV Testing of Pregnant Women and Newborns. (1990). HIV infection, pregnant women, and newborns: A policy proposal for information and testing. *Journal of the American Medical Association, 264,* 2416-2420.

American Psychological Association. (1987, July 27). *Behavioral issues in pediatric AIDS/HIV infection.* Testimony before the House Select Committee on Narcotics and Control.

American Psychological Association. (1991, August). *Legal liability related to confidentiality and the prevention of HIV transmission.* Resolution adopted by the Council of Representatives at its meeting in San Francisco.

American Psychological Association, Committee for the Protection of Human Participants in Research. (1985, July). Ethical issues in research on AIDS. *APA Monitor,* p. 26. (Reprinted in *IRB,* 1986, *8*(4), 8-10, and *Journal of Homosexuality,* 1986, *13*(1), 93-101)

Americans With Disabilities Act of 1990, Pub. L. 101-336, 104 Stat. 327.

Ammann, A. J. (1988). Immunopathogenesis of pediatric acquired immunodeficiency syndrome. *Journal of Perinatology, 8,* 154-159.

Ammann, A. J. (1990). Pediatric AIDS. In P. T. Cohen, M. A. Sande, & P. A. Volberding (Eds.), *The AIDS knowledge base* (chap. 8, pp. 1-10). Waltham, MA: Medical Publishing Group.

Andiman, W. A., & Modlin, J. F. (1991). Vertical transmission. In P. A. Pizzo & C. M. Wilfert (Eds.), *Pediatric AIDS: The challenge of HIV infection in infants, children, and adolescents* (pp. 140-155). Baltimore, MD: Williams & Wilkins.

Antoni, M. H., Schneiderman, N., Fletcher, M. A., Goldstein, D. A., Ironson, G., & Laperriere, A. (1990). Psychoneuroimmunology and HIV-1. *Journal of Consulting and Clinical Psychology, 58,* 38-49.

Bacchetti, P., & Moss, A. R. (1989). Incubation period of AIDS in San Francisco. *Nature, 338,* 251-253.

Bailey, W. A. (1991, April). AIDS prevention: A sad state of affairs. *Psychology & AIDS Exchange,* p. 2.

Baldwin, J. D., & Baldwin, J. I. (1988). Factors affecting AIDS-related sexual risk-taking behavior among college students. *Journal of Sex Research, 25,* 181-196.

Balis, F. M., & Poplack, D. G. (1991). Drug development and clinical pharmacology. In P. A. Pizzo & C. M. Wilfert (Eds.), *Pediatric AIDS: The challenge of HIV infection in infants, children, and adolescents* (pp. 457-477). Baltimore, MD: Williams & Wilkins.

Barker, L. F., Brown, L. S., Des Jarlais, D. C., Friedman, S. R., Hubbard, R. L., Lindenbaum, S., Miller, H. G., Newmeyer, J. A., & Stryker, J. (1989). AIDS and IV drug use. In C. F. Turner, H. G. Miller, & L. E. Moses (Eds.), *AIDS: Sexual behavior and intravenous drug use.* Washington, DC: National Academy Press.

Barnes, D. M. (1991, September). Too hot to handle: Sex, AIDS, and politics. *Journal of NIH Research,* 10.

Barrett, M. E., Simpson, D., & Lehman, W. (1988). Behavioral changes of adolescents in drug abuse intervention programs. *Journal of Consulting and Clinical Psychology, 44,* 462-463.

Batchelor, W. F. (1988). AIDS 1988: The science and the limits of science. *American Psychologist, 43,* 853-858.

Beaman, M. L., & Strader, M. K. (1989). STD patients' knowledge about AIDS and attitudes toward condom use. *Journal of Community Health Nursing, 6,* 155-164.

Becker, M. H., & Joseph, J. (1988). AIDS and behavioral changes to reduce risk: A review. *American Journal of Public Health, 78,* 394-410.

Bell, T., & Hein, K. (1984). The adolescent and sexually transmitted diseases. In K. Holmes, P. A. Mardh, P. S. Sparling, & P. J. Wiesner (Eds.), *Sexually transmitted diseases.* New York: McGraw-Hill.

Belman, A. L., Diamond, G., Dickson, D., Horoupian, D., Llena, J., Lantos, G., & Rubinstein, A. (1988). Pediatric acquired immunodeficiency syndrome: Neurologic syndrome. *American Journal of Diseases of Children, 142*, 29-35.

Belman, A. L., Ultman, M. H., Horoupian, D., Novick, B., Spiro, A. J., Rubinstein, A., Kurtzberg, D., & Cone-Wesson, B. (1985). Neurological complications in infants and children with acquired immune deficiency syndrome (AIDS). *Annals of Neurology, 18*, 560-566.

Berkley, S., Okware, S., & Naamara, W. (1989). Surveillance for AIDS in Uganda. *Acquired Immune Deficiency Syndrome, 3*, 79-85.

Bernstein, L. J., Krieger, B., Novick, B., Sicklick, M. J., & Rubinstein, A. (1985). Bacterial infection in the acquired immunodeficiency syndrome of children. *Pediatric Infectious Disease, 4*, 472-475.

Biggar, R. J. (1986). The AIDS problem in Africa. *Lancet, 1*, 79-83.

Blanche, S., Rouzioux, C., Moscato, M. G., Veber, F., Mayaux, M., Jacomet, C., Tricoire, J., Deville, A., Vial, M., Firtion, G., de Crepy, A., Douard, D., Robin, M., Courpotin, C., Ciraru-Vigneron, N., Le Deist, F., Griscelli, C., & HIV Infection in Newborns French Collaborative Study Group. (1989). A prospective study of infants born to women seropositive for human immunodeficiency virus type 1. *New England Journal of Medicine, 320*, 1643-1648.

Bliwise, N. G., Grade, M., Irish, T. M., & Ficarrotto, T. J. (1991). Measuring medical and nursing students' attitudes toward AIDS. *Health Psychology, 10*, 289-295.

Blumenfield, M., Smith, P. J., Milazzo, J., Seropian, S., & Wormser, G. P. (1987). Survey of attitudes of nurses working with AIDS patients. *General Hospital Psychiatry, 9*, 58-63.

Board of Education v. Cooperman, 105 N.J. 587, 523 A.2d 655 (1987).

Boston City Hospital to open nation's first residence for terminally ill children with AIDS. (1986, December 1). *AIDS Record*, p. 5.

Botvin, G. J., Baker, E., Botvin, E. M., Filazzola, A. D., & Millman, R. B. (1984). Prevention of alcohol misuse through the development of personal and social competence: A pilot study. *Journal of Studies on Alcohol, 45*, 550-552.

Bronfenbrenner, U. (1979). *The ecology of human development: Experiments by nature and design.* Cambridge, MA: Harvard University Press.

AU: adolescence or adolescents

Brook, J. S., Whiteman, M., & Gordon, A. S. (1983). Stages of drug use in adolescence: Personality, peer, and family correlates. *Developmental Psychology, 19*, 269-277.

Brooks, M. K. (1990). *Legal issues for alcohol and other drug use prevention and treatment programs serving high-risk youth* (OSAP Technical Report No. 2). Washington, DC: Government Printing Office.

Brooks-Gunn, J., Boyer, C. B., & Hein, K. (1988). Preventing HIV infection and AIDS in children and adolescents: Behavioral research and intervention strategies. *American Psychologist, 43*, 958-964.

Brooks-Gunn, J., & Furstenberg, F. F. (1989). Adolescent sexual behavior. *American Psychologist, 44*, 249-257.

Brouwers, P., Belman, A., & Epstein, L. (1991). Central nervous system involvement: Manifestations and evaluation. In P. A. Pizzo & C. M. Wilfert (Eds.), *Pediatric*

AIDS: The challenge of HIV infection in infants, children, and adolescents (pp. 318-335). Baltimore, MD: Williams & Wilkins.

Brouwers, P., Moss, H., Wolters, P., Eddy, J., Balis, F., Poplack, D. G., & Pizzo, P. A. (1990). Effect of continuous-infusion zidovudine therapy on neuropsychologic functioning in children with symptomatic human immunodeficiency virus infection. Journal of Pediatrics, 117, 980-985.

Brown, L. K., & Fritz, G. K. (1988). Children's knowledge and attitudes about AIDS. Journal of the Academy of Child and Adolescent Psychiatry, 27, 504-508.

Brown, L. K., Nassau, J. H., & Levy, V. (1990). "What upsets me most about AIDS is . . .": A survey of children and adolescents. AIDS Education and Prevention, 2, 296-304.

Brunk, M., Henggeler, S. W., & Whelan, J. P. (1987). A comparison of multisystemic therapy and parent training in the brief treatment of child abuse and neglect. Journal of Consulting and Clinical Psychology, 55, 311-318.

Bryson, Y., & Arvin, A. (1991). Herpes group virus infection in HIV-1-infected infants, children, and adolescents. In P. A. Pizzo & C. M. Wilfert (Eds.), Pediatric AIDS: The challenge of HIV infection in infants, children, and adolescents (pp. 245-265). Baltimore, MD: Williams & Wilkins.

Cal. Health & Safety Code § 199.27 (West 1990). (Enacted in 1988)

Campos, P. E., Brasfield, T. L., & Kelly, J. A. (1989). Psychology training related to AIDS: Survey of doctoral graduate programs and predoctoral internship programs. Professional Psychology: Research and Practice, 20, 214-220.

Castro, K. G., Lieb, S., Jaffe, H. W., Narkunas, J. P., Calisher, C. H., Bush, T. J., & Witte, J. J. (1988). Transmission of HIV in Belle Glade, Florida: Lessons for other communities in the United States. Science, 239, 193-197.

Centers for Disease Control. (1982). Update on acquired immune deficiency syndrome (AIDS)—U.S. Morbidity and Mortality Weekly Report, 31, 507-514.

Centers for Disease Control. (1984). Acquired immunodeficiency syndrome (AIDS) in persons with hemophilia. Morbidity and Mortality Weekly Report, 33, 589.

Centers for Disease Control. (1985a). Revision of the case definition of acquired immunodeficiency syndrome for national reporting, United States. Morbidity and Mortality Weekly Report, 34, 373-374.

Centers for Disease Control. (1985b). Recommendations for assisting in the prevention of perinatal transmission of human T-lymphotropic virus type III/lymphadenopathy-associated virus and acquired immunodeficiency syndrome. Morbidity and Mortality Weekly Report, 34, 721-726.

Centers for Disease Control. (1985c). Education and foster care of children infected with human T-lymphotropic virus type III/lymphadenopathy-associated virus. Morbidity and Mortality Weekly Report, 34, 517-521.

Centers for Disease Control. (1987a). Classification system for human immunodeficiency virus (HIV) in children under 13 years of age. Morbidity and Mortality Weekly Report, 36, 225-230, 235-236.

Centers for Disease Control. (1987b). Public health service guidelines for counseling and antibody testing to prevent HIV infection and AIDS. Morbidity and Mortality Weekly Report, 36, 509-515.

Centers for Disease Control. (1987c). U.S. Department of Health and Human Services: Revising the CDC surveillance case definition of acquired immunodeficiency syndrome. *Morbidity and Mortality Weekly Report, 36*(Suppl. 18), 35-55.

Centers for Disease Control. (1987d). Human immunodeficiency virus infection transmitted from an organ donor screened for HIV antibody: North Carolina. *Morbidity and Mortality Weekly Report, 36*, 306-308, 314-315.

Centers for Disease Control. (1989, December). *HIV/AIDS surveillance report.* Atlanta, GA: Author.

Centers for Disease Control. (1990a). Estimates of HIV prevalence and projected AIDS cases: Summary of a workshop, October 31-November 1, 1989. *Morbidity and Mortality Weekly Report, 39*, 110-119.

Centers for Disease Control. (1990b). AIDS in women, United States. *Morbidity and Mortality Weekly Report, 39*, 845-846.

Centers for Disease Control. (1990c). HIV/AIDS surveillance report. *Morbidity and Mortality Weekly Report, 39*, 1-22.

Centers for Disease Control. (1990d). HIV-1 infection and artificial insemination with processed semen. *Morbidity and Mortality Weekly Report, 39*, 249-256.

Centers for Disease Control. (1990e). Possible transmission of human immunodeficiency virus to a patient during an invasive dental procedure. *Morbidity and Mortality Weekly Report, 39*, 489-493.

Centers for Disease Control. (1990f). Update: Acquired immunodeficiency syndrome—United States, 1989. *Morbidity and Mortality Weekly Report, 39*, 81-86.

Centers for Disease Control. (1991a). *HIV/AIDS surveillance report: Year-end edition, 1990.* Washington, DC: U.S. Department of Health and Human Services.

Centers for Disease Control. (1991b). Premarital sexual experience among adolescent women, United States, 1970-1988. *Morbidity and Mortality Weekly Report, 39*, 929-932.

Centers for Disease Control. (1991c). Update: Transmission of HIV infection during an invasive dental procedure, Florida. *Morbidity and Mortality Weekly Report, 40*, 21-28.

Chaisson, R. E., Moss, A., Onishi, R., Osmond, D., & Carlson, J. R. (1987). Human immunodeficiency virus infection in heterosexual intravenous drug users in San Francisco. *American Journal of Public Health, 77*, 169-172.

Chorba, T. L., Berkelman, R. L., Safford, S. K., Gibbs, N. P., & Hull, H. F. (1990). Mandatory reporting of infectious diseases by clinicians. *Morbidity and Mortality Weekly Report, 39*, 1-10.

Christiansen, B. A., Smith, G. T., Roehling, P. V., & Goldman, M. S. (1989). Using alcohol expectancies to predict adolescent drinking behavior after one year. *Journal of Consulting and Clinical Psychology, 57*, 93-99.

Chu, S., Buehler, J. W., & Berkelman, R. L. (1990). Impact of the human immunodeficiency virus epidemic on mortality in women of reproductive age, United States. *Journal of the American Medical Association, 264*, 225-229.

Clark, S. D., Zabin, L. S., & Hardy, J. B. (1984). Sex, contraception, and parenthood: Experience and attitudes among urban black young men. *Family Planning Perspectives, 16*, 77-82.

Coates, T. J., Stall, R., Mandel, J. S., Boccellari, A., Sorenson, J. L., Morales, E. F., Morin, S. F., Wiley, J. A., & McKusick, L. (1987). AIDS: A psychosocial research agenda. *Annals of Behavioral Medicine, 9*, 21-28.

Cook, T. D., & Campbell, D. T. (1979). *Quasi-experimentation: Design and analysis issues for field settings.* Boston: Houghton Mifflin.

Crawford, I., Humfleet, G., Ribordy, S. C., Ho, F. C., & Vickers, V. L. (1991). Stigmatization of AIDS patients by mental health professionals. *Professional Psychology: Research and Practice, 22*, 357-361.

Dawes, R. M. (1988, June). *Measurement models for rating and comparing risks: The context of AIDS.* Paper presented at a conference on Health Services Research Methods: A Focus on AIDS, Tucson. (Cited in C. F. Turner, H. G. Miller, & L. E. Moses, *AIDS: Sexual behavior and intravenous drug use.* Washington, DC: National Academy Press.)

Dawson, D. A. (1988). *AIDS knowledge, misinformation, and perceived risk: Data from the 1987 National Health Interview Survey.* Hyattsville, MD: Division of Health Interview Statistics, National Center for Health Statistics.

Dawson, D. A., & Hardy, A. M. (1989). AIDS knowledge and attitudes of black Americans: Provisional data from the 1988 National Health Interview Survey. *NCHS Advance Data* (No. 165). Hyattsville, MD: Division of Health Interview Statistics, National Center for Health Statistics.

Del. Code Ann. tit. 16, 1203(a)(8) (Cum. Supp. 1990).

DeLoye, G. J., Henggeler, S. W., & Daniels, C. M. (1992). *Developmental and family correlates of children's knowledge and attitudes regarding AIDS.* Manuscript submitted for publication.

Dembo, R., Washburn, M., Wish, E. D., Yeung, H., Getreu, A., Berry, E., & Blount, W. R. (1987). Heavy marijuana use and crime among youths entering a juvenile detention center. *Journal of Psychoactive Drugs, 19*, 47-56.

Department of Health and Human Services, *Additional Protections for Children Involved as Participants in Research,* 45 CFR pt. 46D (1991a).

Department of Health and Human Services, *Additional Protections Pertaining to Research, Development, and Related Activities Involving Fetuses, Pregnant Women, and Human In Vitro Fertilization,* 45 CFR pt. 46B (1991b).

Department of Health and Human Services, Division of Maternal and Child Health. (1987, April). *Children with HIV infection and their families.* Surgeon General's workshop at Children's Hospital, Philadelphia.

Des Jarlais, D. C., Chamberland, M. E., Yancovitz, S. R., Weinberg, P., & Friedman, S. R. (1984). Heterosexual partners: A large risk group for AIDS. *Lancet, 2*, 1346-1347.

Des Jarlais, D. C., & Friedman, S. R. (1987a). Target groups for preventing AIDS among intravenous drug users. *Journal of Applied Social Psychology, 17*, 251-268.

Des Jarlais, D. C., & Friedman, S. R. (1987b). HIV infection among intravenous drug users: Epidemiology and risk reduction. *AIDS, 1*, 67-76.

Des Jarlais, D. C., & Friedman, S. R. (1988). The psychology of preventing AIDS among intravenous drug users: A social learning conceptualization. *American Psychologist, 43*, 865-870.

Des Jarlais, D. C., Friedman, S. R., & Hopkins, W. (1985). Risk reduction for the acquired immunodeficiency syndrome among intravenous drug users. *Annals of Internal Medicine, 103*, 755-759.

DiClemente, R. J., Forrest, K. A., Mickler, S., et al. (1990). College students' knowledge and attitudes about AIDS and changes in HIV-preventive behaviors. *AIDS Education and Prevention, 2*, 201-212.

DiClemente, R. J., Zorn, J., & Temoshok, L. (1986). Adolescents and AIDS: A survey of knowledge, attitudes and beliefs about AIDS in San Francisco. *American Journal of Public Health, 76*, 1443-1445.

Di Maria, H., Courpotin, C., Rouzioux, C., Cohen, D., Rio, D., & Boussin, F. (1986). Transplacental transmission of human immunodeficiency virus. *Lancet, 2*, 215-216.

District 27 Community School Board v. Board of Education, 130 Misc. 2d 398, 502 N.Y.S. 325 (Sup. Ct. 1986).

Doe v. Belleville Public School District, 672 F. Supp. 342 (S.D. Ill. 1987).

Dolan, R., Corber, S., & Zacour, R. (1990). A survey of knowledge and attitudes with regard to AIDS among grade 7 and 8 students in Ottawa-Carleton. *Canadian Journal of Public Health, 81*, 135-138.

Douard, D., Perel, Y., Michaeu, M., Contraires, B., Bonici, J. F., & Fleury, H. J. A. (1989). Perinatal HIV infection: Longitudinal study of 22 children (clinical and biological follow-up). *Journal of Acquired Immune Deficiency Syndrome, 2*, 212-213.

Drucker, E., & Vermund, S. (1987). A method for estimating HIV seroprevalence rates in urban areas with high rates of IV drug abuse: The case of the Bronx. *Abstracts of the Third International Conference on Acquired Immunodeficiency Syndrome.* Washington, DC: U.S. Department of Health and Human Services and the World Health Organization.

Edwards, J. R., Ulrich, P. P., Weintrub, P. S., Cowan, M. J., Levy, J. A., Wara, D. W., & Vyas, G. N. (1989). Polymerase chain reaction compared with concurrent viral cultures for rapid identification of human immunodeficiency virus among high-risk infants and children. *Journal of Pediatrics, 115*, 200-203.

Elliott, D. S., Ageton, S. S., Huizinga, D., Knowles, B. A., & Canter, R. J. (1983). *The prevalence and incidence of delinquent behavior: 1976-1980.* Boulder, CO: Behavioral Research Institute.

Elliott, D. S., Huizinga, D., & Ageton, S. S. (1985). *Explaining delinquency and drug use.* Beverly Hills, CA: Sage.

English, A. (1987). Adolescents and AIDS: Legal and ethical questions multiply. *Youth Law News, 8*(6), 1-6.

Epstein, L. G., Goudsmit, J., Paul, D. A., Morrison, S. H., Connor, E. M., Oleske, J. M., & Holland, B. (1987). Expression of human immunodeficiency virus in cerebrospinal fluid of children with progressive encephalopathy. *Annals of Neurology, 21*, 397.

Epstein, L. G., Sharer, L. R., & Goudsmit, J. (1988). Neurological and neuropathological features of human immunodeficiency virus infection in children. *Annals of Neurology, 23*(Suppl.), 19-23.

Epstein, L. G., Sharer, L. R., Oleske, J. M., Connor, E. M., Goudsmit, J., Bagdon, L., Robert-Guroff, M., & Koenigsberger, M. R. (1986). Neurologic manifestations of human immunodeficiency virus infection in children. *Pediatrics, 78,* 678.

European Collaborative Study. (1988). Mother-to-child transmission of HIV infection. *Lancet, 2,* 1039-1042.

Eyster, M. E. (1991). Transfusion and coagulation factor acquired disease. In P. A. Pizzo & C. M. Wilfert (Eds.), *Pediatric AIDS: The challenge of HIV infection in infants, children, and adolescents* (pp. 22-37). Baltimore, MD: Williams & Wilkins.

Falloon, J., Eddy, J., Wiener, L., & Pizzo, P. A. (1989). Human immunodeficiency virus in children. *Journal of Pediatrics, 114,* 1-30.

Fischl, M. A., Dickinson, G. M., Scott, G. B., Klimas, N., Fletcher, M. A., & Parks, W. (1987). Evaluation of heterosexual partners, children, and household contacts of adults with AIDS. *Journal of the American Medical Association, 257,* 640-644.

Fischl, M. A., Richman, D. D., Hansen, N., Collier, A. C., Carey, J. T., Para, M. F., Hardy, W. D., Dolin, R., Powderly, W. G., Allan, J. D., Wong, B., Merigan, T. C., McAuliffe, V. J., Hyslop, N. E., Rhame, F. S., Balfour, H. H., Spector, S. A., Volberding, P., Pettinelli, C., Anderson, J., & AIDS Clinical Trial Group. (1990). The safety and efficacy of zidovudine in the treatment of subjects with mildly symptomatic human immunodeficiency virus type 1 (HIV) infection. *Annals of Internal Medicine, 112,* 727-737.

Fisher, J. D. (1988). Possible effects of reference group-based social influence on AIDS-risk behavior and AIDS prevention. *American Psychologist, 43,* 914-920.

Fisher, J. D., & Misovich, S. J. (1990). Evolution of college students' AIDS-related behavioral responses, attitudes, knowledge, and fear. *AIDS Education and Prevention, 2,* 322-337.

Flora, J. A., & Thoresen, C. E. (1988). Reducing the risk of AIDS in adolescents. *American Psychologist, 43,* 965-970.

Flora, J. A., & Thoresen, C. E. (1989). Components of a comprehensive strategy for reducing the risk of AIDS in adolescents. In V. M. Mays, G. W. Albee, & S. F. Schneider (Eds.), *Primary prevention of AIDS.* Newbury Park, CA: Sage.

Flynn, N. M., Jain, S., Harper, S., Bailey, V., Anderson, R., & Acuna, G. (1987). *Sharing of paraphernalia in intravenous drug users (IVDU): Knowledge of AIDS is incomplete and doesn't affect behavior.* Paper presented at the Third International Conference on AIDS, Washington, DC.

Forrest, J. D., & Silverman, J. (1989). What public school teachers teach about preventing pregnancy, AIDS, and sexually transmitted diseases. *Family Planning Perspectives, 21,* 65-72.

Friedland, G. H., & Klein, R. S. (1987). Transmission of the human immunodeficiency virus. *New England Journal of Medicine, 317,* 1125-1135.

Friedland, G. H., Saltzman, B. R., Rogers, M. F., Kahl, P. A., Lesser, M. L., Mayers, M. M., & Klein, R. S. (1986). Lack of transmission of HTLV-III/LAV infection to household contacts of patients with AIDS or AIDS-related complex with oral candidiasis. *New England Journal of Medicine, 314,* 344-349.

Fullilove, R. E., Fullilove, M. T., Bowser, B. P., & Gross, S. A. (1990). Risk of sexually transmitted disease among black adolescent crack users in Oakland and San Francisco, California. *Journal of the American Medical Association, 263,* 851-855.

Furstenberg, F. F., Moore, K. A., & Peterson, J. L. (1985). Sex education and sexual experience among adolescents. *American Journal of Public Health, 75,* 1331-1332.

Futterman, D., & Hein, K. (1991). Medical management of adolescents. In P. A. Pizzo & C. M. Wilfert (Eds.), *Pediatric AIDS: The challenge of HIV infection in infants, children, and adolescents* (pp. 546-560). Baltimore, MD: Williams & Wilkins.

Gagnon, J. H., Lindenbaum, S., Martin, J. L., May, R. M., Menken, J., Turner, C. R., & Zabin, L. S. (1989). Sexual behavior and AIDS. In C. F. Turner, H. G. Miller, & L. E. Moses (Eds.), *AIDS: Sexual behavior and intravenous drug use.* Washington, DC: National Academy Press.

Garcia, S. A., & Keilitz, I. (1991). Involuntary civil commitment of drug dependent persons with special reference to pregnant women. *Mental and Physical Disability Law Reporter, 15,* 418-437.

Gardner, W. (1991, June 17). *Adolescents and AIDS: Epidemiology and prevention.* Testimony before the House Select Committee on Children, Youth, and Families. Washington, DC.

Gardner, W., & Herman, J. (1990). Adolescents' AIDS risk taking: A rational choice perspective. In W. Gardner, S. G. Millstein, & B. L. Wilcox (Eds.), *Adolescents in the AIDS epidemic* (pp. 17-34). San Francisco: Jossey-Bass.

Garmezy, N. (1987). Stress, competence, and development: Continuities in the study of schizophrenic adults, children vulnerable to psychopathology, and the search for stress-resilient children. *American Journal of Orthopsychiatry, 57,* 159-174.

Gayle, H. D., & D'Angelo, L. J. (1991). Epidemiology of AIDS and HIV infection in adolescents. In P. A. Pizzo & C. M. Wilfert (Eds.), *Pediatric AIDS: The challenge of HIV infection in infants, children, and adolescents* (pp. 38-50). Baltimore, MD: Williams & Wilkins.

Gayle, J. A., Selik, R. M., & Chu, S. Y. (1990). Surveillance for AIDS and HIV infection among black and Hispanic children and women of childbearing age, 1981-1989. *Morbidity and Mortality Weekly Report, 39,* 23-30.

General Accounting Office. (1991). *ADMS block grant: Women's set-aside does not assure drug treatment for pregnant women* (Report No. GAO/HRD-91-80). Washington, DC: Author.

Gerbert, B., Maguire, B., Badner, V., Altman, D., & Stone, G. (1989). Fear of AIDS: Issues for health professional education. *AIDS Education and Prevention, 1,* 39-52.

Gibbs, J. T. (1986). Psychosocial correlates of sexual attitudes and behaviors in urban early adolescent females: Implications for intervention. *Journal of Social Work & Human Sexuality, 5,* 81-97.

Ginzburg, H. M., French, J., Jackson, J., Hartsock, P. I., MacDonald, M. G., & Weiss, S. H. (1986). Health education and knowledge assessment of HTLV-III diseases among intravenous drug users. *Health Education Quarterly, 13,* 373-382.

Glover v. Eastern Nebraska Office of Retardation, 686 F. Supp. 243 (D.Neb. 1988).

Goodwin, M. P., & Roscoe, B. (1988). AIDS: Students' knowledge and attitudes at a midwestern university. *Journal of American College Health, 36,* 214-222.

Gostin, L. O. (1990a). The AIDS Litigation Project: A national review of court and human rights commission decisions. Part I: The social impact of AIDS. *Journal of the American Medical Association, 263,* 1961-1970.

Gostin, L. O. (1990b). The AIDS Litigation Project: A national review of court and human rights commission decisions. Part II: Discrimination. *Journal of the American Medical Association, 263,* 2086-2093.

Gottlieb, N. H., Vacalis, T. D., Palmer, D. R., & Conlon, R. T. (1988). AIDS-related knowledge, attitudes, behaviors, and intentions among Texas college students. *Health Education Research, 3,* 67-73.

Gray, J. N. (1989). Pediatric AIDS research: Legal, ethical, and policy influences. In J. M. Seibert & R. A. Olson (Eds.), *Children, adolescents, and AIDS* (pp. 179-227). Lincoln: University of Nebraska Press.

Gray, J. N., & Melton, G. B. (1985). The law and ethics of psychosocial research on AIDS. *Nebraska Law Review, 64,* 637-688.

Greenwald, J., Melton, G. B., & Nellis, M. (1991). *Psychosocial obstacles to safer sex among university undergraduates.* Unpublished manuscript.

Grossman, M. (1988). Children with AIDS. In I. Corless & M. Pittman-Lindeman (Eds.), *AIDS: Principles, practices, and politics* (pp. 167-173). Washington, DC: Hemisphere.

Grossman, M. (1990). Special problems in the child with AIDS. In M. A. Sande & P. A. Volberding (Eds.), *The medical management of AIDS* (2nd ed., pp. 385-397). Philadelphia: W. B. Saunders.

Guinan, M. E., & Hardy, A. (1987). Epidemiology of AIDS in women in the United States—1981 through 1986. *Journal of the American Medical Association, 257,* 2039-2042.

Gwinn, M., George, R., Hannon, H., Hoff, R., Pappaioanou, M., & Novello, A. (1990). Estimates of HIV seroprevalence in childbearing women and incidence of HIV infection in infants—United States. *Abstracts of the Sixth International Conference on Acquired Immunodeficiency Syndrome.* Washington, DC: U.S. Department of Health and Human Services and the World Health Organization.

Halebsky, M. A. (1987). Adolescent alcohol and substance abuse: Parent and peer effects. *Adolescence, 22,* 961-967.

Hamilton, D. P. (1991). Hints emerge from the Gallo probe. *Science, 253,* 728-729.

Hartwig, A. C., & Eckland, J. D. (1991). Policy issues concerning HIV-positive children: State education officials' opinions. *AIDS & Public Policy Journal, 6,* 91-97.

Haseltine, W. A. (1989). Development of antiviral drugs for the treatment of AIDS: Strategies and prospects. *Journal of Acquired Immune Deficiency Syndrome, 2,* 311-334.

Haseltine, W. A., & Wong-Staal, F. (1988). The molecular biology of the AIDS virus. *Scientific American, 259,* 52-62.

Haverkos, H. W. (1987). Factors associated with the pathogenesis of AIDS. *Journal of Infectious Diseases, 156,* 251-257.

Haverkos, H. W., & Smeriglio, V. L. (1991). Cofactors and HIV. In P. A. Pizzo & C. M. Wilfert (Eds.), *Pediatric AIDS: The challenge of HIV infection in infants, children, and adolescents* (pp. 75-81). Baltimore, MD: Williams & Wilkins.

Hayes, C. D. (1987). *Risking the future: Adolescent sexuality, pregnancy, and childbearing.* Washington, DC: National Academy Press.

Hayes, C. E., Sharp, E. S., & Miner, K. R. (1989). Knowledge, attitudes, and beliefs of HIV seronegative women about AIDS. *Journal of Nurse-Midwifery, 34,* 291-295.

Heagarty, M. C. (1991). Pediatric acquired immunodeficiency syndrome, poverty, and national priorities. *American Journal of Diseases of Children, 145,* 527-528.

Hegarty, J. D., Abrams, E. J., Hutchinson, V. E., et al. (1988). The medical care costs of human immunodeficiency virus-infected children in Harlem. *Journal of the American Medical Association, 260,* 1901-1905.

Hein, K. (1987a). AIDS in adolescents: A rationale for concern. *New York State Journal of Medicine, 87,* 290-295.

Hein, K. (1987b). The use of therapeutics in adolescence. *Journal of Adolescent Health Care, 8,* 8-35.

Hein, K. (1989). Commentary on adolescent acquired immunodeficiency syndrome: The next wave of the human immunodeficiency virus epidemic? *Journal of Pediatrics, 114,* 144-149.

Hein, K. (1991). Fighting AIDS in adolescents. *Issues in Science and Technology, 7(3),* 67-72.

Henggeler, S. W. (1989). *Delinquency in adolescence.* Newbury Park, CA: Sage.

Henggeler, S. W. (1991). Multidimensional causal models of delinquent behavior. In R. Cohen & A. Siegel (Eds.), *Context and development.* Hillsdale, NJ: Lawrence Erlbaum.

Henggeler, S. W., & Borduin, C. M. (1990). *Family therapy and beyond: A multisystemic approach to treating the behavior problems of children and adolescents.* Pacific Grove, CA: Brooks/Cole.

Henggeler, S. W., Melton, G. B., & Smith, L. (in press). Family preservation using multisystemic therapy: An effective alternative incarcerating serious juvenile offenders. *Journal of Consulting and Clinical Psychology.*

Henggeler, S. W., Rodick, J. D., Borduin, C. M., Hanson, C. L., Watson, S. M., & Urey, J. R. (1986). Multisystemic treatment of juvenile offenders: Effects on adolescent behavior and family interaction. *Developmental Psychology, 22,* 132-141.

Herek, G. M., & Glunt, E. K. (1988). An epidemic of stigma: Public reactions to AIDS. *American Psychologist, 43,* 886-891.

Herold, E. S., Fisher, W. A., Smith, E. A., & Yarber, W. A. (1990). Sex education and the prevention of STD/AIDS and pregnancy among youths. *Canadian Journal of Public Health, 81,* 141-145.

Hill, W. C., Bolton, V., & Carlson, J. R. (1987). Isolation of acquired immunodeficiency syndrome virus from the placenta. *American Journal of Obstetrics and Gynecology, 157,* 10-11.

Hingson, R. W., Strunin, L., & Berlin, B. M. (1990). Acquired immunodeficiency syndrome transmission: Changes in knowledge and behaviors among teenagers, Massachusetts statewide surveys, 1986-1988. *Pediatrics, 85,* 24-29.

Hingson, R. W., Strunin, L., Berlin, B. M., & Heeren, T. (1990). Beliefs about AIDS, use of alcohol and drugs, and unprotected sex among Massachusetts adolescents. *American Journal of Public Health, 80,* 295-299.

Ho, D. D., Pomerantz, R. J., & Kaplan, J. C. (1987). Pathogenesis of infection with human immunodeficiency virus. *New England Journal of Medicine, 317,* 278-286.

Hodgson v. Minnesota, 110 S.Ct. 2926 (1990).

Hofferth, S. L., Kahn, J. R., & Baldwin, W. (1987). Premarital sexual activity among U.S. teenage women over the past three decades. *Family Planning Perspectives, 19,* 46-53.

Howe, E. G. (1990). Societal and clinical approaches to preventing pediatric AIDS: Some ethical considerations. *AIDS & Public Policy Journal, 5,* 9-16.

Huba, G. J., Wingard, J. A., & Bentler, P. M. (1980). Applications of a theory of drug use to prevention programs. *Journal of Drug Education, 10,* 25-38.

Hughes, W. T. (1991). Pneumocystis carinii pneumonia. In P. A. Pizzo & C. M. Wilfert (Eds.), *Pediatric AIDS: The challenge of HIV infection in infants, children, and adolescents* (pp. 288-298). Baltimore, MD: Williams & Wilkins.

Human Immunodeficiency Virus Services Act of 1989, Tex. Rev. Civ. Stat. Ann. arts. 4419b-4 to 4419b-6 (Vernon Cum. Supp. 1991).

Hutto, C., Parks, W. P., Lai, S., Mastrucci, M. T., Mitchell, C., Munoz, J., Prapido, E., Master, I. M., & Scott, G. B. (1991). A hospital-based prospective study of perinatal infection with human immunodeficiency virus type 1. *Journal of Pediatrics, 118,* 347-353.

Imagawa, D. T., Lee, M. H., Wolinsky, S. M., Sano, K., Morales, F., Kwok, S., Sninsky, J. J., Nishanian, R. G., Giorgi, J., Fahey, J. L., Dudley, J., Visscher, B. R., & Detels, R. (1989). Human immunodeficiency virus type 1 infection in homosexual men who remain seronegative for prolonged periods. *New England Journal of Medicine, 320,* 1458-1462.

Imperato, P. J., Feldman, J. G., Nayeri, K., & DeHovitz, J. A. (1988). Medical students' attitudes towards caring for patients with AIDS in a high incidence area. *New York State Journal of Medicine, 88,* 223-227.

Ingold, F. R., & Ingold, S. (1989). The effects of the liberalization of syringe sales on the behavior of intravenous drug users in France. *Bulletin on Narcotics, 41,* 67-81.

Institute of Medicine. (1991). *HIV screening of pregnant women and newborns.* Washington, DC: National Academy Press.

Iowa Code Ann. § 141.22(6) (West 1989b). (Enacted in 1988)

Iowa Code Ann. § 141.9(2) (West 1989a). (Enacted in 1988)

Italian Multicentre Study. (1988). Epidemiology, clinical features, and prognostic factors in paediatric HIV infection. *Lancet, 2,* 1043-1046.

Jackson, J., & Rotkiewicz, L. (1987). *A coupon program: AIDS education and drug treatment.* Paper presented at the Third International Conference on AIDS, Washington, DC.

Jaffe, L. R., Seehaus, M., Wagner, C., & Leadbeater, B. J. (1988). Anal intercourse and knowledge of acquired immunodeficiency syndrome among minority-group female adolescents. *Journal of Pediatrics, 112,* 1005-1007.

Jeffries, D. J. (1989). Targets for antiviral therapy of human immunodeficiency virus infection. *Journal of Infection, 18,* 5-13.

Jessor, R., & Jessor, S. L. (1977). *Problem behavior and psychosocial development: A longitudinal study of youth*. New York: Academic Press.

Johnson v. State, 578 So.2d 419 (Fla. App. 5th Dist. 1991).

Johnson, C. A., Pentz, M. A., Weber, M. D., Dwyer, J. H., Baer, N., MacKinnon, D. P., Hansen, W. B., & Flay, B. R. (1990). Relative effectiveness of comprehensive community programming for drug abuse prevention with high-risk and low-risk adolescents. *Journal of Consulting and Clinical Psychology, 58,* 447-456.

Johnson, E. M. (1987). Substance abuse and women's health. *Public Health Reports, 1,* 42-48.

Johnson, J. P., Nair, P., Hines, S. E., Seiden, S. W., Alger, L., Revie, D. R., O'Neil, K. M., & Hebel, R. (1989). Natural history and serologic diagnosis of infants born to human immunodeficiency virus-infected women. *American Journal of Diseases in Children, 143,* 1147-1153.

Johnson, S. D. (1987). Factors related to intolerance of AIDS victims. *Journal for the Scientific Study of Religion, 26,* 105-110.

Jones, J. L., Wykoff, R. F., Hollis, S. L., Longshore, S. T., Gamble, W. B., Jr., & Gunn, R. A. (1990). Partner acceptance of health department notification of HIV exposure, South Carolina. *Journal of the American Medical Association, 264,* 1284-1286.

Joseph, J. G., Montgomery, S., Kirscht, J., Kessler, R., Ostrow, D., Wortman, C., Brian, K., Eller, M., & Eshlem, S. (1987). Perceived risk of AIDS: Assessing the behavioral and psychosocial consequences in a cohort of gay men. *Journal of Applied Psychology, 17,* 231-250.

Joshi, N. P., & Scott, M. (1988). Drug use, depression, and adolescents. *Pediatric Clinics of North America, 35,* 275-288.

Kandel, D. B. (1980). Drug and drinking behavior among youth. *Annual Review of Sociology, 6,* 235-285.

Karan, L. D. (1989). AIDS prevention and chemical dependence treatment needs of women and their children. *Journal of Psychoactive Drugs, 21,* 395-399.

Katzman, E. M., Mulholland, M., & Sutherland, E. M. (1988). College students and AIDS: A preliminary survey of knowledge, attitudes, and behavior. *Journal of American College Health, 37,* 127-130.

Kazak, A. E. (1989). Families of chronically ill children: A systems and social-ecological model of adaptation and challenge. *Journal of Consulting and Clinical Psychology, 57,* 25-30.

Kazdin, A. E. (1987). *Conduct disorders in childhood and adolescence*. Newbury Park, CA: Sage.

Keeling, R. P. (1988). Effective responses to AIDS in higher education. *Thought & Action: The NEA Higher Education Journal, 4,* 5-22.

Kegeles, S. M., Adler, N. E., & Irwin, C. E. (1988). Sexually active adolescents and condoms: Changes over one year in knowledge, attitudes, and use. *American Journal of Public Health, 78,* 460-461.

Kelly, J. A., St. Lawrence, J. S., Smith, S., Hood, H. V., & Cook, D. J. (1987a). Medical students' attitudes toward AIDS and homosexual patients. *Journal of Medical Education, 62,* 549-556.

Kelly, J. A., St. Lawrence, J. S., Smith, S., Jr., Hood, H. V., & Cook, D. J. (1987b). Stigmatization of AIDS patients by physicians. *American Journal of Public Health, 77*, 789-791.

Kemper, K., & Forsyth, B. (1988). Medically unnecessary hospital use in children seropositive for human immunodeficiency virus. *Journal of the American Medical Association, 260*, 1906-1909.

Kiecolt-Glaser, J. K., & Glaser, R. (1987). Psychosocial moderators of immune function. *Annals of Behavioral Medicine, 9*, 16-20.

King, N. J., & Gullone, E. (1990). Fear of AIDS: Self-reports of Australian children and adolescents. *Psychological Reports, 66*, 245-246.

Knapp, S., & VandeCreek, L. (1990). Application of the duty to protect to HIV-positive patients. *Professional Psychology: Research and Practice, 21*, 161-166.

Kolata, G. (1991, August 25). U.S. rule on fetal studies hampers research on AZT. *The New York Times*, p. Y13.

Krasinski, K., Borkowsky, W., Bonk, S., Lawrence, R., & Chandwani, S. (1988). Bacterial infections in human immunodeficiency virus infected children. *Pediatric Infectious Disease, 7*, 323-328.

Krasinski, K., Borkowsky, W., & Holzman, R. S. (1989). Prognosis of human immunodeficiency virus infection in children and adolescents. *Pediatric Infectious Disease, 8*, 216-220.

La Greca, A. M. (1988). Adherence to prescribed medical regimens. In D. K. Routh (Ed.), *Handbook of pediatric psychology* (pp. 299-320). New York: Guilford.

Landers, D. V., & Sweet, R. L. (1991). Prospects for prenatal diagnosis of fetal HIV infection. In P. A. Pizzo & C. M. Wilfert (Eds.), *Pediatric AIDS: The challenge of HIV infection in infants, children, and adolescents* (pp. 175-183). Baltimore, MD: Williams & Wilkins.

Landesman, S., Minkoff, H., Hollman, S., McCalla, S., & Sijn, O. (1987). Serosurvey of human immunodeficiency virus infection in parturients. *Journal of the American Medical Association, 258*, 2701-2703.

Lapointe, N., Michaud, J., Pekovic, D., Chausseau, J. P., & Dupuy, J. M. (1985). Transplacental transmission of HTLV-III virus. *New England Journal of Medicine, 312*, 1325-1326.

Laure, F., Courgnaud, V., Rouzioux, C., Blanche, S., Veber, F., Burgard, M., Jacomet, C., Griscelli, C., & Brechot, C. (1988). Detection of HIV-1 DNA in infants and children by means of polymerase chain reaction. *Lancet, 2*, 538-541.

Leukefeld, C. G., Battjes, R. J., & Amsel, Z. (1990). Community prevention efforts to reduce the spread of AIDS associated with intravenous drug abuse. *AIDS Education and Prevention, 2*, 235-243.

Levin, B. W., Driscoll, J. M., Jr., & Fleischman, A. R. (1991). Treatment choice for infants in the neonatal intensive care unit at risk for AIDS. *Journal of the American Medical Association, 265*, 2976-2981.

Lewin, C., & Williams, R. J. (1988). Fear of AIDS: The impact of public anxiety in young people. *British Journal of Psychiatry, 153*, 823-824.

Lewis, C., Battistich, V., & Schaps, E. (1990). School-based primary prevention: What is an effective program? In W. Gardner, S. G. Millstein, & B. L. Wilcox (Eds.), *Adolescents in the AIDS epidemic* (pp. 35-59). San Francisco: Jossey-Bass.

Lewis, C. E., Freeman, H. E., & Corey, C. R. (1987). AIDS-related competence of California's primary care physicians. *American Journal of Public Health, 77,* 795-799.

Lewis, C. E., & Montgomery, K. (1990). The HIV-testing policies of U.S. hospitals. *Journal of the American Medical Association, 264,* 2764-2767.

Lewis, D., Das, N. K., Hoppner, C. L., & Jencks, M. (1991). A program of support for AIDS research in the social/behavioral sciences. *MIRA, 5*(3), 2-5.

Lewitt, E. M., Coate, D., & Grossman, M. (1981). The effects of government regulation of teenage smoking. *Journal of Law and Economics, 24,* 545-569.

Lifson, A. R. (1988). Do alternate modes for transmission of human immunodeficiency virus exist? A review. *Journal of the American Medical Association, 259,* 1353-1356.

Link, R. N., Feingold, A. R., Charap, M. H., Freeman, K., & Shelov, S. P. (1988). Concerns of medical and pediatric house officers about acquiring AIDS from their patients. *American Journal of Public Health, 78,* 455-459.

Liss, M. B. (1989). The schooling of children with AIDS: The development of policies. In J. M. Seibert & R. A. Olson (Eds.), *Children, adolescents, and AIDS* (pp. 93-117). Lincoln: University of Nebraska Press.

Lusher, J. M., & Warrier, I. (1991). Medical management of children and adolescents with hemophilia. In P. A. Pizzo & C. M. Wilfert (Eds.), *Pediatric AIDS: The challenge of HIV infection in infants, children, and adolescents* (pp. 531-545). Baltimore, MD: Williams & Wilkins.

Magrab, P. R., & Wohlford, P. (Eds.). (1990). *Clinical training in psychology: Improving psychological services for children and adolescents with severe mental disorders.* Washington, DC: American Psychological Association.

Manning, D. T., & Balson, P. M. (1989). Teenagers' beliefs about AIDS education and physicians' perceptions about them. *Journal of Family Practice, 29,* 173-177.

Manning, D. T., Barenberg, N., Gallese, L., & Rice, J. C. (1989). College students' knowledge and health beliefs about AIDS: Implications for education and prevention. *Journal of American College Health, 37,* 254-259.

Manoff, S. B., Gayle, H. D., Mays, M. A., & Rogers, M. F. (1989). Acquired immunodeficiency syndrome in adolescents: Epidemiology, prevention and public health issues. *Pediatric Infectious Disease, 8,* 309-314.

Martin, J. M., & Sacks, H. S. (1990). Do HIV-infected children have access to clinical trials of new treatments? *AIDS & Public Policy Journal, 5,* 3-8.

Martinez v. School Board, 861 F.2d 1502 (11th Cir. 1988).

Mata, A. G., & Jorquez, J. S. (1989). Mexican-American intravenous drug users' needle-sharing practices: Implications for AIDS prevention. In V. M. Mays, G. W. Albee, & S. F. Schneider (Eds.), *Primary prevention of AIDS.* Newbury Park, CA: Sage.

Maury, W., Potts, B. J., & Rabson, A. B. (1989). HIV-1 infection of first-trimester and term human placental tissue: A possible mode of maternal-fetal transmission. *Journal of Infectious Diseases, 160,* 583-588.

Mays, V. M. (1989). AIDS prevention in black populations: Methods of a safer kind. In V. M. Mays, G. W. Albee, & S. F. Schneider (Eds.), *Primary prevention of AIDS.* Newbury Park, CA: Sage.

Mays, V. M., & Cochran, S. D. (1987). Acquired immunodeficiency syndrome and black Americans: Special psychosocial issues. *Public Health Reports, 102,* 224-231.

Mays, V. M., & Cochran, S. D. (1988). Issues in the perception of AIDS risk and risk reduction activities by black and Hispanic/Latina women. *American Psychologist, 43,* 949-957.

McClure, M. O., & Weiss, R. A. (1987). Human immunodeficiency virus and related viruses. In M. S. Gottlieb (Ed.), *Current topics in AIDS: Vol. 1* (pp. 95-117). New York: John Wiley.

McCutchan, J. A. (1990). Virology, immunology, and clinical course of HIV infection. *Journal of Consulting and Clinical Psychology, 58,* 5-12.

McDermott, R. J., Hawkins, M. J., Moore, J. R., & Cittadino, S. K. (1987). AIDS awareness and information sources among selected university students. *Journal of American College Health, 35,* 222-226.

McKinney, R. E., Jr., Maha, M. A., Connor, E. M., Feinberg, J., Scott, G. B., Wulfsohn, M., McIntosh, K., Borkowsky, W., Modlin, J. F., Weintrub, P., O'Donnell, K., Gelber, R. D., Rogers, G. K., Lehrman, S. N., Wilfert, C. M., & Protocol 043 Study Group. (1991). A multicenter trial of oral zidovudine in children with advanced human immunodeficiency virus disease. *New England Journal of Medicine, 324,* 1018-1025.

McKusick, L., Horstman, W., & Coates, T. J. (1985). AIDS and sexual behavior reported by gay men in San Francisco. *American Journal of Public Health, 75,* 493-496.

McNamara, J. G. (1989). Immunologic abnormalities in infants infected with human immunodeficiency virus. *Seminars in Perinatology, 13,* 35-43.

Medicare Catastrophic Coverage Act of 1988, Pub. L. 100-360, 102 Stat. 683.

Melton, G. B. (1983). Minors and privacy: Are legal and psychological concepts compatible? *Nebraska Law Review, 62,* 455-493.

Melton, G. B. (1987). Children, politics, and morality: The ethics of child advocacy. *Journal of Clinical Child Psychology, 16,* 357-367.

Melton, G. B. (1988a). Adolescents and prevention of AIDS. *Professional Psychology: Research and Practice, 19,* 403-408.

Melton, G. B. (1988b). Ethical and legal issues in AIDS-related practice. *American Psychologist, 43,* 941-947.

Melton, G. B. (1989a). Ethical and legal issues in research and intervention. *Journal of Adolescent Health Care, 10,* 36S-44S.

Melton, G. B. (1989b). Public policy and private prejudice: Psychology and law on gay rights. *American Psychologist, 44,* 933-940.

Melton, G. B. (1990). Certificates of confidentiality under the Public Health Service Act: Strong protection but not enough. *Violence and Victims, 5,* 67-71.

Melton, G. B., & Ehrenreich, N. S. (in press). Ethical and legal issues in mental health services for children. In C. E. Walker & M. C. Roberts (Eds.), *Handbook of clinical child psychology* (2nd ed.). New York: Plenum.

Melton, G. B., & Gray, J. N. (1988). Ethical dilemmas in AIDS research: Individual privacy and public health. *American Psychologist, 43,* 60-64.

Melton, G. B., & Hargrove, D. S. (in press). *Planning mental health services for children and youth.* New York: Guilford.

Mich. Comp. Laws Ann. § 333.5131 (West Cum. Supp. 1991).

Miller, H. G., Turner, C. F., & Moses, L. E. (1990). *AIDS: The second decade.* Washington, DC: National Academy Press.

Mills, C. J., & Noyes, H. L. (1984). Patterns and correlates of initial and subsequent drug use among adolescents. *Pediatric Clinics of North America, 33,* 275-288.

Mitchell, J. L., & Heagarty, M. (1991). Special considerations for minorities. In P. A. Pizzo & C. M. Wilfert (Eds.), *Pediatric AIDS: The challenge of HIV infection in infants, children, and adolescents* (pp. 704-713). Baltimore, MD: Williams & Wilkins.

Mnookin, R. H., & Weisberg, K. (1989). *Child, family, and state* (2nd ed.). Boston: Little, Brown.

Mo. Ann. Stat. § 191.688(1)(1) (Vernon Cum. Supp. 1991). (Enacted in 1988)

Mok, J. Q., DeRossi, A., Ades, A. E., Giaquinto, C., Grosch-Worner, I., & Peckham, C. S. (1987). Infants born to mothers seropositive for human immunodeficiency virus. *Lancet, 1,* 1164-1168.

Mondanaro, J. (1987). Strategies for AIDS prevention: Motivating health behavior in drug dependent women. *Journal of Psychoactive Drugs, 19,* 143-149.

Morrison, D. M. (1985). Adolescent contraceptive behavior: A review. *Psychological Bulletin, 98,* 538-568.

Mott, F. (1985). *Evaluation of fertility data and preliminary analytical results from the 1983 survey of the National Longitudinal Surveys of Work Experience of Youth* (Technical Report). Columbus: Ohio State University, Center for Human Resource Research.

Munoz, A., Wang, M., Bass, S., Taylor, J. M. G., Kingsley, L. A., Chimiel, J. S., Polk, B. F., & Multicenter AIDS Cohort Study Group. (1989). Acquired immunodeficiency syndrome (AIDS)-free time after seroconversion in homosexual men. Multicenter AIDS Cohort Study Group. *American Journal of Epidemiology, 130,* 530-539.

Murphy-Brown, V., & Sullivan, M. (1991, August). *Attitudes about services for substance abusing parents and their children.* Paper presented at the Summer Institute on Mental Health Law, Lincoln, NE.

Nadal, D., Hunziker, V. A., Schupbach, J., Wetzel, J. C., Tomasik, Z., Jendis, J. B., Fanconi, A., & Seger, R. A. (1989). Immunologic evaluation in the early diagnosis of prenatal or perinatal HIV infection. *Archives of Diseases in Children, 64,* 662-669.

Nadel, M. V. (1990, May 3). *AIDS education: Gaps in coverage still exist.* Testimony on behalf of the General Accounting Office before the Senate Committee on Governmental Affairs.

Neaigus, A., Sufian, M., Friedman, S. R., Goldsmith, D. S., Stepherson, B., Mota, P., Pascal, J., & Des Jarlais, D. C. (1990). Effects of outreach intervention on risk reduction among intravenous drug users. *AIDS Education and Prevention, 2,* 253-271.

Neb. Rev. Stat. § 43-2102 (Reissue 1988).

Neb. Rev. Stat. § 71-504 (Reissue 1990).

Nemechek, P. M. (1991). Anabolic steroid users: Another potential risk group for HIV infection. *Journal of the American Medical Association, 325,* 357.

Nev. Rev. Stat. Ann. § 441A.220(4) (Michie 1989).

N.J. Stat. Ann. §§ 26.5C-5 and 26.5C-13 (West Cum. Supp. 1991). (Enacted in 1989)

N.Y. Pub. Health Law § 2780(5) (McKinney Cum. Supp. 1991). (Enacted in 1988)

New York State Association for Retarded Children v. Carey, 612 F.2d 644 (2d Cir. 1979).

Nolan, K. (1990). AIDS and pediatric research. *Evaluation Review, 14,* 464-481.

N.C. Gen. Stat. 130A-148(h) (1990).

Novello, A. C., Wise, P. H., Willoughby, A., & Pizzo, P. A. (1989). Final report of the United States Department of Health and Human Services Secretary's Work Group on pediatric human immunodeficiency virus infection and disease: Content and implications. *Pediatrics, 84,* 547-555.

Novick, L. F., Berns, D., Stricof, R., Stevens, R., Pass, K., & Wethers, J. (1989). HIV seroprevalence in newborns in New York state. *Journal of the American Medical Association, 261,* 1745-1750.

O'Donnell, L., O'Donnell, C. R., Pleck, J. H., Snarey, J., & Rose, R. M. (1987). Psychosocial responses of hospital workers to acquired immune deficiency syndrome (AIDS). *Journal of Applied Social Psychology, 17,* 269-285.

Oetting, E. R., & Beauvais, R. (1990). Adolescent drug use: Findings of national and local surveys. *Journal of Consulting and Clinical Psychology, 58,* 385-394.

Oetting, E. R., Edwards, R. W., & Beauvais, F. (1989). Drugs and Native-American youth. In B. Segal (Ed.), *Perspectives on adolescent drug abuse.* Binghamton, NY: Haworth.

Oleske, J., Minnefor, A., Cooper, R., Thomas, K., Cruz, A., Ahdieh, H., Guerrero, I., Joshi, V. V., & Desposito, F. (1983). Immune deficiency syndrome in children. *Journal of the American Medical Association, 249,* 2345-2349.

Oliva, G. E., Rutherford, G. W., Grossman, M., Shalwitz, J., English, A., Taylor, F., & Werdegar, D. (1988). Guidelines for the control of human immunodeficiency virus infection in adolescents. *Western Journal of Medicine, 148,* 586-589.

Olson, R. A., Huszti, H. C., Mason, P. J., & Seibert, J. M. (1989). Pediatric AIDS/HIV Infection: An emerging challenge to pediatric psychology. *Journal of Pediatric Psychology, 14,* 1-21.

O'Reilly, K. R., & Aral, S. O. (1985). Adolescence and sexual behavior. *Journal of Adolescent Health Care, 6,* 262-270.

Orlandi, M. A. (1986). Community-based substance abuse prevention: A multicultural perspective. *Journal of School Health, 56,* 394-401.

Osgood, D. W., & Wilson, J. K. (1989). *Covariation among health-compromising behaviors in adolescence.* Report to the U.S. Congress, Office of Technology Assessment, Washington, DC. (NTIS No. PB 91-154 377/AS)

Osmond, D. (1990a). Numbers and demographic characteristics of U.S. cases. In P. T. Cohen, M. A. Sande, & P.A. Volberding (Eds.), *The AIDS knowledge base* (chap. 1, pp. 1-4). Waltham, MA: Medical Publishing Group.

Osmond, D. (1990b). AIDS in Africa. In P. T. Cohen, M. A. Sande, & P.A. Volberding (Eds.), *The AIDS knowledge base* (chap. 4, pp. 1-10). Waltham, MA: Medical Publishing Group.

Ou, C. Y., Kwok, S., Mitchell, S. W., Mack, D. H., Sninsky, J. J., Krebs, J. W., Feorino, P., Warfield, D., & Schochetman, G. (1988). DNA amplification for direct detection of HIV-1 in DNA of peripheral blood mononuclear cells. *Science, 239,* 295-297.

Overby, K. J., Lo, B., & Litt, I. F. (1989). Knowledge and concerns about acquired immune-deficiency syndrome and their relationship to behavior among adolescents with hemophilia. *Pediatrics, 83,* 204-210.

Oxtoby, M. J. (1988). Human immunodeficiency virus and other viruses in human milk: Placing the issues in broader perspective. *Pediatric Infectious Disease, 7,* 825-835.

Oxtoby, M. J. (1991). Perinatally acquired HIV infection. In P. A. Pizzo & C. M. Wilfert (Eds.), *Pediatric AIDS: The challenge of HIV infection in infants, children, and adolescents* (pp. 3-21). Baltimore, MD: Williams & Wilkins.

Palmore v. Sidoti, 466 U.S. 433 (1984).

Parks, W. P., & Scott, G. B. (1987). An overview of pediatric AIDS: Approaches to diagnosis and outcome assessment. In S. Broder (Ed.), *AIDS: Modern concepts and therapeutic challenges* (pp. 245-262). New York: Marcel Dekker.

Parry, J. W. (1991). Using the Reporter to research key Americans With Disabilities Act provisions. *Mental and Physical Disability Law Reporter, 15,* 16-19.

Pelton, S. I., & Klein, J. O. (1991). Bacterial diseases in infants and children with infections due to HIV. In P. A. Pizzo & C. M. Wilfert (Eds.), *Pediatric AIDS: The challenge of HIV infection in infants, children, and adolescents* (pp. 199-208). Baltimore, MD: Williams & Wilkins.

Peterson, J. L., & Marin, G. (1988). Issues in the prevention of AIDS among black and Hispanic men. *American Psychologist, 43,* 871-877.

Phipps v. Saddleback Valley Unified School District, No. 4747981 (Orange County, Calif., Super. Ct. 1986).

Piot, P., Plummer, F. A., Mhalu, F. S., Chin, J., & Mann, J. M. (1988). AIDS: An international perspective. *Science, 239,* 573-579.

Pizzo, P. A. (1990). Pediatric AIDS: Problems within problems. *Journal of Infectious Diseases, 161,* 316-325.

Pizzo, P. A., Eddy, J., Falloon, J., Balis, F. M., Murphy, R. F., Moss, H., Wolters, P., Browers, P., Jarosinski, P., Rubin, M., Broder, S., Yarchoan, R., Brunetti, A., Maha, M., Nusinoff-Lehrman, S., & Poplack, D. G. (1988). Effect of continuous intravenous infusion of zidovudine (AZT) in children with symptomatic HIV infection. *New England Journal of Medicine, 319,* 889-896.

Pizzo, P. A., & Wilfert, C. M. (1991). Treatment considerations for children with HIV infection. In P. A. Pizzo & C. M. Wilfert (Eds.), *Pediatric AIDS: The challenge of HIV infection in infants, children, and adolescents* (pp. 478-494). Baltimore, MD: Williams & Wilkins.

Pomerance, L. M., & Shields, J. J. (1989). Factors associated with hospital workers' reactions to the treatment of persons with AIDS. *AIDS Education and Prevention, 1,* 184-193.

Price, J. H., Desmond, S., & Kukulka, G. (1985). High school students' perceptions and misperceptions of AIDS. *Journal of School Health, 55,* 107-109.

Price, M. E. (1989, August 7). Searching for a new paradigm. *National Law Journal*, pp. 13-14, 16-17.

Quay, H. C. (Ed.). (1987). *Handbook of juvenile delinquency.* New York: John Wiley.

Quinn, T. C., Ruff, A., & Halsey, N. (1991). Special considerations for developing nations. In P. A. Pizzo & C. M. Wilfert (Eds.), *Pediatric AIDS: The challenge of HIV infection in infants, children, and adolescents* (pp. 714-744). Baltimore, MD: Williams & Wilkins.

Ralph, N., & Spigner, C. (1986). Contraceptive practices among female heroin addicts. *American Journal of Public Health, 76*, 1016-1017.

Ranki, A., Valle, S. L., & Krohn, M. (1987). Long latency precedes overt seroconversion in sexually transmitted human immunodeficiency-virus infection. *Lancet, 2*, 589-593.

Ray v. School District, 666 F. Supp. 1524 (M.D. Fla. 1987).

Rehabilitation Act of 1973, 29 U.S.C. §§ 701-709, 720-724, 730-732, 740-741, 750, 760-764, 770-776, 780-787, & 790-794 (1988).

Reid, D. A. (1988). Knowledge of school-children about the acquired immune deficiency syndrome. *Journal of the Royal College of General Practitioners, 38*, 509-510.

Reinisch, J. M., Sanders, S. A., & Ziemba-Davis, M. (1988). The study of sexual behavior in relation to the transmission of human immunodeficiency virus. *American Psychologist, 43*, 921-927.

Remafedi, G. (1987a). Adolescent homosexuality: Psychosocial and medical implications. *Pediatrics, 79*, 331-337.

Remafedi, G. J. (1987b). Homosexual youth: A challenge to contemporary society. *Journal of the American Medical Association, 258*, 222-225.

Remafedi, G. J. (1988). Preventing the sexual transmission of AIDS during adolescence. *Journal of Adolescent Health Care, 9*, 139-143.

Rhodes, J. E., & Jason, L. A. (1988). *Preventing substance abuse among children and adolescents.* New York: Pergamon.

Rhodes, J. E., & Jason, L. A. (1990). A social stress model of substance abuse. *Journal of Consulting and Clinical Psychology, 58*, 395-401.

Richwald, G. A., Sekler, J. C., Kitimbo, D. W., & Friedland, J. M. (1989). Public health students' knowledge of AIDS: Implications for HIV-related training needs. *AIDS Education and Prevention, 1*, 89-95.

Robertson v. Granite City Community Unit School District No. 9, 684 F. Supp. 1002 (S.D. Ill. 1988).

Robertson, J. R., Bucknall, A. B., & Welsby, P. D. (1986). Epidemic of AIDS related virus (HTLV-III/LAV) infection among IV drug abusers. *British Medical Journal, 292*, 527-529.

Rogers, M. (1989). Perinatal infection. In R. A. Kaslow & D. P. Francis (Eds.), *The epidemiology of AIDS: Expression, occurrence, and control of human immunodeficiency virus type 1 infection* (pp. 231-241). New York: Oxford University Press.

Rogers, M. F., Ou, C., Kilbourne, B., & Schochetman, G. (1991). Advances and problems in the diagnosis of HIV infection in infants. In P. A. Pizzo & C. M. Wilfert (Eds.), *Pediatric AIDS: The challenge of HIV infection in infants, children, and adolescents* (pp. 159-174). Baltimore, MD: Williams & Wilkins.

Rogers, M. F., Ou, C., Rayfield, M., Thomas, P. A., Schoenbaum, E. E., Abrams, E., Krasinski, K., Selwyn, P. A., Moore, J., Kaul, A., Grimm, K. T., Bamji, M., Schochetman, G. & New York City Collaborative Study of Maternal HIV Transmission and Montefiore Medical Center HIV Perinatal Transmission Study Group. (1989). Use of the polymerase chain reaction for early detection of the proviral sequences of human immunodeficiency virus in infants born to seropositive mothers. *New England Journal of Medicine, 320,* 1649-1654.

Rogers, M. F., Thomas, P. A., Starcher, E. T., Noa, M. C., Bush, T. J., & Jaffe, H. W. (1987). Acquired immunodeficiency syndrome in children: Report of the Centers for Disease Control national surveillance, 1982-1985. *Pediatrics, 79,* 1008-1014.

Rosenberg, Z. F., & Fauci, A. S. (1991). Immunopathology and pathogenesis of HIV infection. In P. A. Pizzo & C. M. Wilfert (Eds.), *Pediatric AIDS: The challenge of HIV infection in infants, children, and adolescents* (pp. 82-94). Baltimore, MD: Williams & Wilkins.

Rotheram-Borus, M., Koopman, C., Haignere, C., & Davies, M. (1991). Reducing HIV sexual risk behaviors among runaway adolescents. *Journal of the American Medical Association, 266,* 1237-1241.

Royse, D., & Birge, B. (1987). Homophobia and attitudes towards AIDS patients among medical, nursing, and paramedical students. *Psychological Reports, 61,* 867-870.

Royse, D., Dhooper, S. S., & Hatch, L. R. (1987). Undergraduate and graduate students' attitudes toward AIDS. *Psychological Reports, 60,* 1185-1186.

Rubinstein, A., Sicklick, M., Gupta, A., Bernstein, L., Klein, N., Rubinstein, E., Spigland, I., Fruchter, L., Litman, N., Lee, H., & Hollander, M. (1983). Acquired immunodeficiency with reversed T4/T8 ratios in infants born to promiscuous and drug addicted mothers. *Journal of the American Medical Association, 249,* 2350-2356.

Ruiz, P. (1985). Cultural barriers to effective medical care among Hispanic-American patients. *Annual Review of Medicine, 36,* 63-71.

Rwandan HIV Seroprevalence Study Group. (1989). National community-based serological survey of HIV-1 and other human retrovirus infections in a Central African country. *Lancet, 1,* 941-943.

Ryan White Comprehensive AIDS Resources Emergency Act of 1990, Pub. L. 101-381, 104 Stat. 576.

Ryder, R. W., Nsa, W., Hassig, S. E., Behets, F., Rayfield, M., Ekungola, B., Nelson, A. M., Mulenda, U., Francis, H., Mwandagalirwa, K., Davachi, F., Rogers, M., Nzilambi, N., Greenberg, A., Mann, J., Quinn, T. C., Piot, P., & Curran, J. W. (1989). Perinatal transmission of the human immunodeficiency virus type 1 to infants of seropositive women in Zaire. *New England Journal of Medicine, 320,* 1637-1642.

Sattentau, Q. (1990). Virology of AIDS. In A. Mindel (Ed.), *AIDS: A pocket book of diagnosis and management* (pp. 16-32). Baltimore: Urban & Schwarzenberg.

Schilling, R. F., Schinke, S. P., Nichols, S. E., Zayas, L. H., Miller, S. O., Orlandi, M. A., & Botvin, G. J. (1989). Developing strategies for AIDS prevention research with black and Hispanic drug users. *Public Health Reports, 104,* 2-11.

160 PEDIATRIC AND ADOLESCENT AIDS

Schinke, S. P., Botvin, G. J., Orlandi, M. A., Schilling, R. F., & Gordon, A. N. (1990). African-American and Hispanic-American adolescents, HIV infection, and preventive intervention. *AIDS Education and Prevention, 2*, 305-312.

School Board of Nassau County v. Arline, 480 U.S. 273 (1987).

Schooley, R. T., Merigan, T. C., Gaut, P., Hirsch, M. S., Holodniy, M., Flynn, T., Liu, S., Byington, B. S., Henochowicz, S., Gubish, E., Spriggs, D., Kufe, D., Schindler, J., Dawson, A., Thomas, D., Hanson, D. G., Letwin, B., Liu, T., Gulinello, J., Kennedy, S., Fisher, R., & Ho, D. D. (1990). Recombinant soluble CD4 therapy in patients with the acquired immunodeficiency syndrome and AIDS-related complex: A phase I-II escalating dosage trial. *Annals of Internal Medicine, 112*, 247-253.

Schumacher, R. T., Garrett, P. E., Tegmeier, G. E., & Thomas, D. (1988). Comparative detection of anti-HIV in early HIV seroconversion. *Journal of Clinical Immunoassay, 11*, 130-134.

Scott, G. B., & Hutto, C. (1991). Prognosis in pediatric HIV infection. In P. A. Pizzo & C. M. Wilfert (Eds.), *Pediatric AIDS: The challenge of HIV infection in infants, children, and adolescents* (pp. 187-198). Baltimore, MD: Williams & Wilkins.

Scott, G. B., Hutto, C., Makuch, R. W., Mastrucci, M. T., O'Connor, T., Mitchell, C. D., Trapido, E. J., & Parks, W. P. (1989). Survival in children with perinatally acquired human immunodeficiency virus (HIV) infection: Experience with 172 children in Miami, Florida. *New England Journal of Medicine, 321*, 1791-1796.

Seibert, J. M., Garcia, A., Kaplan, M., & Septimus, A. (1989). Three model pediatric AIDS programs: Meeting the needs of children, families, and communities. In J. M. Seibert & R. A. Olson (Eds.), *Children, adolescents, and AIDS* (pp. 25-60). Lincoln: University of Nebraska Press.

Selik, R. M., Castro, K. G., & Pappaioanou, M. (1988). Racial/ethnic differences in the risk of AIDS in the United States. *American Journal of Public Health, 78*, 1539-1545.

Seltzer, V. L., Rabin, J., & Benjamin, F. (1989). Teenagers' awareness of the acquired immunodeficiency syndrome and the impact of their sexual behavior. *Obstetrics & Gynecology, 74*, 55-59.

Selwyn, P. A., Carter, R. J., Schoenbaum, E. E., Robertson, V. J., Klein, R. S., & Rogers, M. F. (1989). Knowledge of HIV antibody status and decisions to continue or terminate pregnancy among intravenous drug users. *Journal of the American Medical Association, 261*, 3567-3571.

Senturia, Y. D., Ades, A. E., Peckham, C. S., & Giaquinto, C. (1987). Breast feeding and HIV infection. *Lancet, 2*, 400-401.

Shannon, K. M., & Ammann, A. J. (1985). Acquired immune deficiency syndrome in childhood. *Journal of Pediatrics, 106*, 332-342.

Sheridan, K., Coates, T. J., Chesney, M. A., Beck, G., & Morokoff, P. J. (1989). Health psychology and AIDS. *Health Psychology, 8*, 761-765.

Sherman, R. (1991a, May 13). Bioethics debate. *National Law Journal*, pp. 1, 30-31.

Sherman, R. (1991b, October 14). Criminal prosecutions on AIDS growing. *National Law Journal*, pp. 3, 38.

Shrum, J. C., Turner, N. H., & Bruce, K. E. M. (1989). Development of an instrument to measure attitudes toward acquired immune deficiency syndrome. *AIDS Education and Prevention, 1,* 222-230.

Siegel, K., & Gibson, W. C. (1988). Barriers to the modification of sexual behavior among heterosexuals at risk for acquired immunodeficiency syndrome. *New York State Journal of Medicine, 88,* 66-70.

Simkins, L., & Eberhage, M. G. (1984). Attitudes toward AIDS, herpes II, and toxic shock syndrome. *Psychological Reports, 55,* 779-786.

Simkins, L., & Kushner, A. (1986). Attitudes toward AIDS, herpes II, and toxic shock syndrome: Two years later. *Psychological Reports, 59,* 883-891.

Singer, E., Rogers, T. F., & Corcoran, M. (1987). The polls—a report: AIDS. *Public Opinion Quarterly, 51,* 580-595.

Slater, B. R. (1988). Essential issues in working with lesbian and gay male youths. *Professional Psychology: Research and Practice, 19,* 226-235.

Sorensen, R. E. (1973). *Adolescent sexuality in contemporary America: Personal values and sexual behavior.* New York: Abrams.

S.C. Code Ann. § 44-29-135(e) (Law. Co-Op. 1990). (Enacted in 1988)

Sprecher, S., Soumenkoff, G., Puissant, F., & Degueldre, M. (1986). Vertical transmission of HIV in a 15-week fetus. *Lancet, 2,* 288-289.

Srinivasan, A., York, D., & Bohan, C. (1987). Lack of HIV replication in arthropod cells. *Lancet, 1,* 1094-1095.

Stall, R. D., Coates, T. J., & Hoff, C. (1988). Behavioral risk reduction for HIV infection among gay and bisexual men: A review of results from the United States. *American Psychologist, 43,* 878-885.

Stehr-Green, J. K., Bevers, R. H., & Berkelman, R. B. (1990). *Impact for HIV/AIDS on adolescents in the United States* [Abstract]. Sixth International Conference on AIDS: Abstracts, San Francisco, June, 1990.

Stewart, G. J., Tyler, J. P. P., Cunningham, A. L., Barr, J. A., Driscoll, G. L., Gold, J., & Lamont, B. J. (1985). Transmission of human T-cell lymphotropic virus type III (HTLV-III) by artificial insemination by donor. *Lancet, 2,* 581-584.

Stiehm, E. R., & Vink, P. (1991). Transmission of human immunodeficiency virus infection by breast-feeding. *Journal of Pediatrics, 118,* 410-412.

Stiehm, E. R., & Wara, W. A. (1991). Immunology of HIV. In P. A. Pizzo & C. M. Wilfert (Eds.), *Pediatric AIDS: The challenge of HIV infection in infants, children, and adolescents* (pp. 95-112). Baltimore, MD: Williams & Wilkins.

Strader, M. K., & Beaman, M. L. (1989). College students' knowledge about AIDS and attitudes toward condom use. *Public Health Nursing, 6,* 62-66.

Strunin, L., & Hingson, R. (1987). Acquired immunodeficiency syndrome and adolescents: Knowledge, beliefs, attitudes, and behaviors. *Pediatrics, 79,* 825-828.

Strunin, L., Hingson, R., Barry, M. A., & Liebling, L. G. (1988). Should someone with AIDS be allowed to attend school? A statewide survey of adolescents. *AIDS & Public Policy Journal, 3,* 17-20.

Swaim, R. C., Oetting, E. R., Edwards, R. W., & Beauvais, F. (1989). Links from emotional distress to adolescent drug use: A path model. *Journal of Consulting and Clinical Psychology, 57,* 227-231.

Tarasoff v. Regents of the University of California, 131 Cal. Rptr. 14, 551 P.2d 334 (1976).

Task Force on Pediatric AIDS, American Psychological Association. (1989). Pediatric AIDS and human immunodeficiency virus infection: Psychological issues. *American Psychologist, 44,* 258-264.

Teich, N. (1985). Taxonomy of retroviruses. In R. Weiss, N. Teich, H. Varmus, & J. Coffer (Eds.), *RNA tumor viruses* (2nd ed., pp. 26-207). NY: Cold Spring Harbor Laboratory.

Thiry, L., Sprecher-Goldberger, S., Jonckheer, T., Levy, J. A., Van dePerre, P., Henrivaux, P., Cogniauz-LeClerc, J., & Clumeck, N. (1985). Isolation of AIDS virus from cell-free breast milk of three healthy virus carriers. *Lancet, 2,* 891-892.

Thomas v. Atascadero Unified School District, 662 F. Supp. 376 (C.D. Cal. 1987).

Totten, G., Lamb, D. H., & Reeder, G. D. (1990). Tarasoff and confidentiality in AIDS-related psychotherapy. *Professional Psychology: Research and Practice, 21,* 155-160.

Treiber, F. A., Shaw, D., & Malcolm, R. (1987). Acquired immune deficiency syndrome: Psychological impact on health personnel. *Journal of Nervous and Mental Disease, 175,* 496-499.

Triplet, R. G., & Sugarman, D. B. (1987). Reactions to AIDS victims: Ambiguity breeds contempt. *Personality and Social Psychology Bulletin, 13,* 265-274.

Turner, C. F., Miller, H. G., & Moses, L. E. (1989). *AIDS: Sexual behavior and intravenous drug use.* Washington, DC: National Academy Press.

United Nations Convention on the Rights of the Child, U.N. Doc. A/Res/44/25 (1989).

U.S. Advisory Board on Child Abuse and Neglect. (1990). *Child abuse and neglect: Critical first steps in response to a national emergency.* Washington, DC: Government Printing Office

Valdiserri, R. O. (1989). *Preventing AIDS: The design of effective programs.* New Brunswick, NJ: Rutgers University Press.

Valleroy, L. A. (1990, Autumn). Pediatric AIDS and HIV infection in the United States: Recommendations for research, policy, and programs. *Society for Research in Child Development Social Policy Report,* pp. 1-12.

van den Hoek, J. A. R., Coutinho, R. D., van Zadelhoff, A. W., van Haas-Trecht, H. J. A., & Goudsmit, J. (1988). Prevalence, incidence and risk factors of HIV infection among drug users in Amsterdam. *AIDS, 2,* 55-60.

Van Dyke, R. B. (1991). Pediatric human immunodeficiency virus infection and the acquired immunodeficiency syndrome: A health care crisis of children and families. *American Journal of Diseases of Children, 145,* 529-532.

Vogt, M. W., Witt, D. J., Craven, D. E., Byington, R., Crawford, D. F., Schooley, R. T., & Hirsch, M. S. (1986). Isolation of HTLV-III/LAV from cervical secretions of women at risk for AIDS. *Lancet, 1,* 525.

Volberding, P. A., Lagakos, S. W., Koch, M. A., Pettinelli, C., Myers, M. W., Booth, D. K., Balfour, H. H., Reichman, R. C., Bartlett, J. A., Hirsch, M. S., Murphy, R. L., Hardy, W. D., Soeiro, R., Fischl, M. A., Bartlett, J. G., Merigan, T. C., Hyslop, N. E., Richman, D. D., Valentine, F. T., Corey, L., & AIDS Clinical Trials

Groups of the National Institute of Allergy and Infectious Diseases. (1990). Zidovudine in asymptomatic human immunodeficiency virus infection: A controlled trial in persons with fewer than 500 CD4 cells per cubic millimeter. *New England Journal of Medicine, 322,* 941-949.

Voydanoff, P., & Donnelly, B. W. (1990). *Adolescent sexuality and pregnancy.* Newbury Park, CA: Sage.

Wadlington, W. J. (1983). Consent to medical care for minors: The legal framework. In G. B. Melton, G. P. Koocher, & M. J. Saks (Eds.), *Children's competence to consent* (pp. 57-74). New York: Plenum.

Weber, J. N., & Weiss, R. A. (1988). The virology of human immunodeficiency viruses. *British Medical Bulletin, 44,* 20-37.

Weiblen, B. J., Lee, F. K., Cooper, E. R., Landesman, S. H., McIntosh, K., Harris, J. S., Nesheim, S., Mendez, H., Pelton, S. I., Nahmias, A. J., & Hoff, R. (1990). Early diagnosis of HIV infection in infants by detection of IgA HIV antibodies. *Lancet, 1,* 988-990.

Weiblen, B. J., Schumacher, R. T., & Hoff, R. (1990). Detection of IgM and IgA antibodies to HIV-1 after removal of IgG with recombinant protein G. *Journal of Immunological Methods, 126,* 199-204.

Weinbreck, P., Loustaud, P., Denis, F., Vidal, B., Mounier, M., & De Lumley, L. (1998). Postnatal transmission of HIV infection. *Lancet, 1,* 482.

Weiser, B. (1991, July 15). While child suffered, beliefs clashed. *Washington Post,* pp. A1, A6-A7.

Weisman, C. S., Nathanson, C. A., Ensminger, M., Teitelbaum, M. A., Robinson, J. C., & Plichta, S. (1989). AIDS knowledge, perceived risk and prevention among adolescent clients of a family planning clinic. *Family Planning Perspectives, 21,* 213-217.

Wiener, L., & Septimus, A. (1991). Psychosocial consideration and support for the child and family. In P. A. Pizzo & C. M. Wilfert (Eds.), *Pediatric AIDS: The challenge of HIV infection in infants, children, and adolescents* (pp. 577-594). Baltimore, MD: Williams & Wilkins.

Wilber, J. C. (1990). HIV antibody testing: Methodology. In P. T. Cohen, M. A. Sande, & P. A. Volberding (Eds.), *The AIDS knowledge base* (chap. 2, pp. 1-8). Waltham, MA: Medical Publishing Group.

Wilcox, B. L. (1990). Federal policy and adolescent AIDS. In W. Gardner, S. G. Millstein, & B. L. Wilcox (Eds.), *Adolescents in the AIDS epidemic* (pp. 61-70). San Francisco: Jossey-Bass.

Wills, T. A., Baker, E., & Botvin, G. J. (1989). Dimensions of assertiveness: Differential relationships to substance use in early adolescence. *Journal of Consulting and Clinical Psychology, 57,* 473-478.

Wis. Stat. Ann. § 146.025(2)(4) (West Cum. Supp. 1990). (Enacted in 1989)

Wofsy, C. B. (1987). Human immunodeficiency virus infection in women. *Jounal of the American Medical Association, 257,* 2074-2076.

Wong-Staal, F., & Gallo, R. C. (1985). Human T-lymphotropic retroviruses. *Nature, 317,* 395-403.

Wykoff, R. F., Heath, C. W., Jr., Hollis, S. L., Leonard, S. T., Quiller, C. B., Jones, J. L., Artzrouni, M., & Parker, R. L. (1988). Contact tracing to identify human immunodeficiency virus infection in a rural community. *Journal of the American Medical Association, 259*, 3563-3566.

Yolken, R. H., Hart, W., & Perman, J. (1991). Viral infection and gastrointestinal dysfunction in children with HIV infection. In P. A. Pizzo & C. M. Wilfert (Eds.), *Pediatric AIDS: The challenge of HIV infection in infants, children, and adolescents* (pp. 277-287). Baltimore, MD: Williams & Wilkins.

Zelnik, M., & Kantner, J. F. (1980). Sexual activity, contraceptive use and pregnancy among metropolitan-area teenagers: 1971-1979. *Family Planning Perspectives, 12*, 230-237.

Zelnik, M., & Kim, Y. J. (1982). Sex education and its association with teenage sexual activity, pregnancy and contraceptive use. *Family Planning Perspectives, 14*, 117-126.

Zelnik, M., & Shah, F. K., (1983). First intercourse among young Americans. *Family Planning Perspectives, 15*, 64-82.

Ziegler, J. B., Johnson, R. O., Cooper, D. A., & Gold, J. (1985). Postnatal transmission of AIDS-associated retrovirus from mother to infant. *Lancet, 1*, 896-898.

Ziegler, J. B., Stewart, G. J., Penny, R., Stuckey, M., & Good, S. (1988). Breast-feeding and transmission of HIV from mother to infant. *Abstract of the Fourth International Conference on Acquired Immunodeficiency Syndrome*. Washington, DC: U.S. Department of Health and Human Services and the World Health Organization.

Author Index

Link, R. N., 50
Liss, M. B., 128
Litman, N., 9
Litt, I. F., 32
Liu, S., 9.3
Liu, T., 93
Llena, J., 13, 14
Lo, B., 32
Longshore, S. T., 115
Loustad, P., 30
Lusher, J. M., 94

MacDonald, M. G., 70
Mack, D. H., 7
MacKinnon, D. P., 72
Magrab, P. R., 81
Maha, M., 93, 129
Makuch, R. W., 13, 16
Malcolm, R., 50
Mandel, J. S., 132, 135
Mann, J. M., 33, 34
Manning, D. T., 41, 42, 44, 45
Manoff, S. B., 24
Marin, G., 65, 70, 74
Martin, J. L., 53, 54, 57
Martin, J. M., 119
Mason, P. J., 95
Master, I. M., 28
Mastrucci, M. T., 13, 16, 28
Mata, A. G., 68, 76
Maury, W., 29
May, R. M., 53, 54, 57
Mayers, M. M., 33
Mayoux, M., 28
Mays, M. A., 24
Mays, V. M., 65, 74, 75
McAuliffe, V. J., 92
McCalla, S., 33
McClure, M. O., 4
McCutchan, J. A., 4
McDermott, R. J., 42, 44, 45
McIntosh, K., 8, 129
McKinney, R. E., 129
McKusick, L., 89, 132, 135
McNamara, J. G., 5

Melton, G. B., 55, 64, 71, 75, 83, 84, 87, 101, 102, 106, 107, 109, 110, 115, 130
Mendez, H., 8
Menken, J., 53, 54, 57
Merigan, T. C., 92, 93
Mhalu, F. S., 33
Michaeu, M., 15
Michaud, J., 29
Mickler, S., 42, 43, 44, 46, 48, 49, 64
Milazzo, J., 50
Miller, H. G., 68, 69, 70, 72, 76, 77, 78, 81, 82, 84, 86, 88, 125
Miller, S. O., 65, 74, 75
Millman, R. B., 71
Mills, C. J., 71
Miner, K. R., 46
Minkoff, H., 33
Minnefor, A., 9, 129
Misovich, S. J., 42, 46, 64
Mitchell, C. D., 13, 16, 28
Mitchell, J. L., 26
Mitchell, S. W., 7
Mnookin, R. H., 102
Modlin, J. F., 29, 30, 34, 129
Mok, J. Q., 6
Mondanaro, J., 73
Montgomery, K., 114
Montgomery, S., 86
Moore, J., 7
Moore, J. R., 42, 44, 45
Moore, K. A., 60
Morales, F., 11
Morales, E. F., 132, 135
Morin, S. F., 132, 135
Morokoff, P. J., 98
Morrison, D. M., 60
Morrison, S. H., 16
Moscato, M. G., 28
Moses, L. E., 81, 82, 84, 86, 88, 125
Moss, A., 76
Moss, A. R., 11
Moss, H., 93
Mota, P., 77, 78
Mott, F., 53
Mounier, M., 30
Mulenda, U., 34

Subject Index

Abortion, HIV testing and, 108
Acquired immune deficiency syndrome.
  See AIDS
Acting-out behaviors, 55, 56
Adolescents: access to health care, 114;
  AIDS incubation period and, 24-
  25; attitudes toward AIDS, 47-48;
  clinical trials and, 117, 136; condom
  use and, 32, 59, 62; contraceptive
  use and, 58-60; developing countries and, 34; ethical and legal issues and, 105-107; incidence of HIV
  infections, 21, 24-25; IV drug use
  and, 67-69, 138; knowledge about
  AIDS, 40-47; medical management of, 94; modes of transmission
  among, 30-32; needle sharing and,
  84; payment for services and, 116;
  pregnancy and, 58-59; prevention
  programs and, 81-82, 84-86; race/
  ethnicity and, 26; sex education
  and, 60-61, 81-82; sexually transmitted diseases and, 58; special
  populations of, 88

Adolescent sexual behavior, 52-66, 137-
  138; barriers to changing, 64-65; het-
  erosexuality, 55-57; homosexuality,
  57-58; knowledge about AIDS and,
  64-65; since the AIDS epidemic, 61-
  63; substance use and, 72-73
Adoptive parents, confidentiality and,
  112-113
Adults with AIDS, classification scheme
  for, 10
Advocacy groups, 23
Africa, AIDS in, 33-34
African-Americans, 25-26; adolescent
  sexual behavior and, 55-56; contraception and, 59; IV drug use, 74;
  premarital intercourse and, 55; preventive interventions and, 74-75;
  sex education and, 61
AIDS (acquired immune deficiency syndrome): attitudes toward, 37, 47-
  51, 82-83, 136-137, 136-137; clinical
  course of, 134-135; death rates, 2-3;
  definition and classification and, 9-
  11; epidemiology in other nations,

Rational-choice model, risky behavior and, 83
Recombinant CD4 (rCD4), 93-94
Red Cross donors, 21
Regulatory proteins, 4
Rehabilitation Act (1973), 116-117, 121, 128-129
Religion, African-Americans and, 75
Reporting, 19
Reproductive choice, 108
Research, 117; consent for, 107, 108-109; fetuses and, 108-109; foster children and, 119; methodology, 37-40; minors' consent to, 107; noninfected children and adolescents and, 136-138; priorities, 132-138
Research data, retention of identifiable, 101
Respite care, 123
Reverse transcriptase, 3-4
Reverse transcriptase inhibitors, 92
Risk, perceived, 126
Risk behaviors, 46-47, 136; adolescents and, 52; attitudes and, 47; college students and, 64; cultural factors and, 65; rational-choice model and, 83
RNA (ribonucleic acid), 3
Romania, pediatric AIDS and, 34
Runaways, 85, 88, 105, 106, 111
Ryan White Comprehensive AIDS Resources Emergency Act (1990), 127

Safer sex: mixed messages about, 88; negotiating, 65
Saliva, 33, 120
Salmonella, 34
Schools: access to, 120-122; AIDS education in, 82; boycotts of, 126; confidentiality and, 111-112; substance abuse and, 71
Science professionals, credit for advances and, 102
Seat belt use, condom use and, 64

Seizures, 14
Self-esteem, peer group and, 86
Self-reports, of sexual behavior, 53-54
Sepsis, 12
Sex education: adolescents and, 81-82; contraceptive use and, 59; effects of, 60-61
Sexual abstinence, 124
Sexual abuse, transmission via, 113-114
Sexual adventurers, 88
Sexual behavior: adolescents and, 31, 32, 52-66, 72, 137-138; adolescent substance use and, 72-73; college students and, 63; communication problems and, 83; difficulty in alteration of, 87; IV drug users and, 67, 77-78, 87; peer norms and, 84; social cognition and, 63
Sexuality, privacy and, 105
Sexually transmitted diseases (STDs), 41; minors' rights to treatment and, 106; rising incidence of, 25
Sexual partners: college students and, 63; confidentiality and, 115; familiarity with, 56
Sexual transmission, 28
Sinusitis, 12
Social cognition, sexual behavior and, 63
Social context, substance abuse and, 70-72, 74
Social desirability, attitudes toward AIDS and, 39
Social-ecological approach, 96, 137
Social policy, changes in, 89-90
"Social risk," American Medical Association and, 109
Social skills training, 85
Social support, 96
Social systems, adolescent sexual behavior and, 56-57
Socioeconomic status: adolescent sexual behavior and, 57; condom use and, 64
Southeastern states, AIDS prevalence, 27
Soviet Union, pediatric AIDS and, 34

Women of childbearing age, 21, 32-33; AIDS among, 22-24; race/ethnicity and, 25-26

Women's issues, adolescent substance abuse, 72-75

World Health Organization, classification scheme, 11

Young children, symptom presentation in, 11-12

Youth autonomy, state support for, 105

Zidovudine, 92

About the Authors

Scott W. Henggeler is Professor of Psychiatry and Behavioral Sciences at the Medical University of South Carolina. He has published more than 100 journal articles, book chapters, and books, and he is on the editorial board of several journals. Much of his research concerns antisocial behavior in adolescence and the development of effective treatments for such behavior. Recent volumes include *Delinquency in Adolescence* and *Family Therapy and Beyond: A Multisystemic Approach to Treating the Behavior Problems of Children and Adolescents.* He is currently conducting major projects to evaluate the effectiveness of multisystemic therapy with substance-abusing delinquents and with serious juvenile offenders and their multiproblem families.

Gary B. Melton is Carl Adolph Happold Professor of Psychology and Law at the University of Nebraska—Lincoln, where he also directs the Law/Psychology Program and the Center on Children, Families, and the Law. He is vice chair of the U.S. Advisory Board on Child Abuse and Neglect and a member of the American Bar Association Commission on Mental Disability Law. He is a past president of the APA Division of Child, Youth, and Family Services and the American Psychology-Law Society. He has also served as a member of the APA Council of Representatives and the APA Task Force on Psychology and AIDS, and as chair of the APA Committee for the

Protection of Human Participants in Research. In 1985 he received the APA Award for Distinguished Contributions to Psychology in the Public Interest, and in 1992 he received the Nicholas Hobbs Award from the APA Division of Child, Youth, and Family Services. He is the author of nearly 200 publications. Among his books are *Child Advocacy: Psychological Issues and Interventions* and *Psychological Evaluations for the Courts.* He moderates a briefing series for congressional staff, he has testified before committees of Congress several times, and his work has been cited by courts at all levels, including the U.S. Supreme Court. He also has served as a consultant to legislatures, social service agencies, and mental health agencies in several states. He has been a Fulbright scholar at the Norwegian Center for Child Research, and he has been an invited lecturer or consultant in 10 foreign countries.

James R. Rodrigue received his Ph.D. in clinical psychology from Memphis State University in 1989. He completed his internship at the University of Florida Health Sciences Center and now is an Assistant Professor in the Department of Clinical and Health Psychology at the University of Florida. At the University of Florida, he is active in the pediatric and medical psychology consultation-liaison programs and in the training of graduate students, interns, and residents. His research interests are in the areas of pediatric psychology, developmental disabilities, and the application of family-treatment approaches in pediatric health care settings. He has contributed several publications to the pediatric and clinical child literature. In addition to his involvement in clinical, teaching, and research activities, he presently serves as chairman of the APA Division 38 (Health Psychology) Committee on Children and Health, editor of *Update on Children's Health Issues,* a member of the APA Division 12 Task Force on Diversity in Clinical Psychology, and Secretary of the North Florida Chapter of the Florida Psychological Association. He also volunteers his time to conduct community workshops for the American Cancer Society that serve to facilitate the reintegration of children with life-threatening illnesses into the public school system.